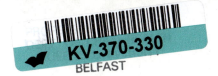

Clinical Investigations in Gastroenterology

ASTRA
GASTROINTESTINAL

Clinical Investigations in Gastroenterology

M.C. Bateson

Consultant Physician and Specialist in Gastroenterology General Hospital, Bishop Auckland, County Durham, UK

and

I.A. . Bouchier

Professor of Medicine, University of Edinburgh, UK

KLUWER ACADEMIC PUBLISHERS
DORDRECHT / BOSTON / LONDON

Distributors

for the United States and Canada: Kluwer Academic Publishers, PO Box 358, Accord Station, Hingham, MA 02018-0358, USA
for all other countries: Kluwer Academic Publishers Group, Distribution Center, PO Box 322, 3300 AH Dordrecht, The Netherlands

British Library Cataloguing in Publication Data

Bateson, Malcolm C. (Malcolm Cedric), 1945 –
    Clinical investigations in gastroenterology.
    1. Man. Gastrointestinal tract. Diagnosis
    I. Title   II. Bouchier, Ian A.D.
    (Ian Arthur Dennis), 1932 –
    616.3'3075

ISBN 0-7462-0103-6

Contents

Preface

This book is a completely up-to-date review of the basic tests available in gastroenterology. It is based on a detailed critical analysis of recently described procedures and the review of more traditional methods; each is assigned its correct place in the modern management of patients. Emphasis is placed on those techniques with which the authors have practical experience. The most useful investigations are indicated in the table of contents by heavy type. Comprehensive references are included to provide information about the selection, performance and interpretation of tests.

The book is designed for trainees and clinicians without special expertise in gastroenterology, as well as being a shelf manual for the gastroenterologist and the staff of gastrointestinal investigation units.

Special thanks are due to the nursing staff of the Day Ward, Bishop Auckland General Hospital; Mr P. Grencis, Medical Photographer; Dr S. Desai, Radiologist; and Amanda Gallagher who typed the manuscript.

Malcolm C. Bateson
Ian A. D. Bouchier
1988

Intubation

The passage of various forms of nasogastric, duodenal and intestinal tubes is basic to many of the diagnostic procedures performed in the gastrointestinal system.

Method

Whenever possible the patient's fullest co-operation should be obtained. If the patient is taking any drugs which might influence the test to be undertaken these should be discontinued.

Before the tube is introduced it is advisable to check that all connections are correct, that the syringe fits snugly on the end of the tube and whether an adaptor is required. The tube is moistened by soaking in water, or lubricated. Many patients cannot, or will not, tolerate the sensation of a tube in the pharyngeal region and a small quantity of local anaesthetic such as 2 per cent lignocaine hydrochloride sprayed on the fauces will prevent a great deal of distress and discomfort. The hazards are minimal and there is no evidence that the agent has any influence on the results of the investigation if it is used sparingly. On the other hand some gastrointestinal functions may be profoundly influenced when the introduction of the tube is accompanied by much hawking, heaving and emotional distress. Thus acid secretion may be inhibited by a technically difficult intubation.

Although most tubes are traditionally introduced via the nose many patients find it more comfortable to swallow a tube by mouth. Sipping water and sucking ice have also been recommended but this may not always be advisable as the aspirate will be diluted and contaminated, and water may be inhaled if the fauces have been anaesthetized. When passing the tube, the patient's neck should be slightly flexed. Most patients find it easier to swallow the tube sitting up, and leaning slightly forward assists passage. It is impossible to swallow when the neck is extended, and flexing the neck guides the tube into the oesophagus.

The passage of tubes through the nose may be difficult and most unpleasant for the patient, and in general it is better to introduce the tube via the mouth. The nasal passages may be deviated or narrowed and many tubes have firm metal ends so that nasal introduction can be awkward, painful and traumatic. The firm indications for introducing a diagnostic tube via the nose

1

include the unconscious patient; the patient who cannot voluntarily co-ordinate swallowing, where sipping water encourages a nasal tube to enter the oesophagus; the patient who refuses to open his mouth; and the patient who persists in biting the tube. The use of the term 'nasogastric' is retained even though the tubes are introduced via the mouth.

If a nasogastric tube enters a bronchus the patient usually coughs, wheezes, or becomes cyanosed, but there are various ways to check the position of the tube: holding the end of the tube against the cheek to feel if air is being exhaled, injecting air via the tube and auscultating over the stomach for a bubbling sound, and testing the aspirated material for acidity.

The problem of the position of a tube need never arise when it is passed for diagnostic purposes because, in general, all small intestinal tubes should be positioned under radiological control. The correct positioning of a tube is usually essential for the accuracy of a diagnostic test. Failure to do this generally invalidates the test. Ideally the position of the tube should be checked radiologically during and at the end of a procedure. The best arrangement is for the procedure room to be equipped with an X-ray image intensifier so that the patient can remain there for the duration of the test. Pre-menopausal women should ideally be examined within 10 days of the onset of menstruation because the radiation dose is considerable.

For gastric secretory studies the tube may be positioned by passing 50-60 cm and then giving the patient 20 ml water to drink. This is aspirated and the tube withdrawn 2.5 cm, and the procedure repeated. This is continued until the highest level at which water can be aspirated is found and the tube taped in position. In this manner radiological monitoring of the tube position is avoided.

The patient can be made more comfortable if the tube is taped to the side of the cheek avoiding the hair, eyebrows and the nose. It also adds to comfort if the external connection is pinned to the garment or pillows so that the tube does not pull on the tape attached to the skin.

It is essential to monitor the aspiration continuously during the investigation. It is quite unsatisfactory to attach the tube to a pump, leave the patient and return to collect the sample at the end of the test period. Ideally, material should be collected by frequent manual aspiration alternating with pump suction, thereby detecting immediately any obstruction to the tube and avoiding mucosa being sucked into the tube because of the development of a negative pressure. If a pump is used its pressure should not be less than 7 mmHg below atmospheric pressure.

The position of the patient will depend to some extent on the test. The usual position is semi-reclining in the supine position, but the patient may incline to left or the right depending on the nature of the procedure.

Tubes

If possible disposable tubes should be employed and used once only.

A great variety of tubes is available and they are generally constructed of plastic. Only a few of the commonly used tubes are mentioned below. Before introduction it is advisable to ascertain whether or not the tube is radio-opaque. Some are not, some are made of X-ray dense material throughout and some radiolucent tubes have metal endpieces to indicate their position. Similar types of tube are made in either radio-opaque or non-radio-opaque material. The majority of tubes are available in varying diameters and in general it is advisable to use the widest diameter compatible with comfort; for plastic tubes No. 14F is the size that is usually convenient. The holes for aspiration should be of a reasonable size, and occasionally it is necessary to enlarge them with a pair of scissors. Tubes with aspiration holes extending too far proximally are valueless; aspiration only occurs if all the holes are under the fluid level and if one is not then only air will be aspirated.

When the duodenum or intestine is being aspirated it is easy for a negative pressure to be established which sucks in the mucosa and blocks the tube. This can be avoided by the use of an extra tube of fine bore attached to the aspirating tube (or incorporated in it) which serves to maintain atmospheric pressure in the bowel.

There are a variety of commercially available tubes, but it is sometimes an advantage to construct a tube for a particular test. This is usually necessary if a very long tube is required for intestinal aspiration. Such tubes are readily made to the required length using either polyethylene or polyvinyl tubing, the latter being preferable because the material is soft and well tolerated by the patient. The tube can be weighted by sealing one end and attaching by a thread a fingercot filled with 2–3 ml of mercury. Vinyl cement or tetrahydrofuran are available for sealing and joining tubes so that double, or multiple, lumen tubes can be constructed. This makes a neat and smooth tube, although multi-lumen tubes may be assembled just as effectively by taping the tubes together with adhesive plaster.

Oesophagus

Any nasogastric tube may be used to aspirate the oesophagus, but short oesophageal tubes are available.

Stomach

The so-called Stomach Tube is a wide-bore tube suitable only for passage via the mouth and only used to wash out the stomach or the oesophagus. It may be used in poisoning, achalasia of the cardia and gastric outflow obstruction.

Many different nasogastric tubes are available for diagnostic work. A 120 cm Salen sump tube (Figure 1) with an inbuilt air-leak channel and a continuous radio-opaque strip is especially convenient when X-ray screening is used. The proximal end is compatible with a bladder syringe, which avoids the need for adaptors. Alternatives are the Ryle's Tube, with a weighted end, and the Levin tube.

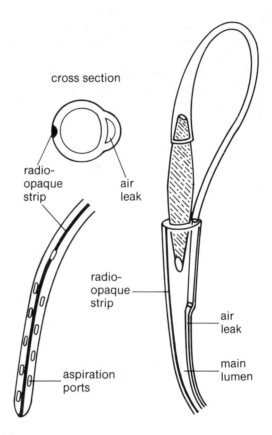

cross section

radio-
opaque
strip

air
leak

radio-
opaque
strip

air
leak

main
lumen

aspiration
ports

Figure 1 Salen sump tube

Duodenum

The diagnostic tubes described above are frequently used for duodenal in-tubation.

When aspirating the duodenum it is often necessary to exclude gastric secretions. For this two separate nasogastric tubes may be swallowed, but bilumen duodenal tubes are also available. Widely used is the Dreiling tube, although homemade multi-lumen tubes are easily constructed. When correctly positioned, these have one set of aspirating holes situated in the stomach antrum and another in the second or third parts of the duodenum. Although it may be more comfortable for the patient to retain a single tube, it is sometimes difficult to be certain that a single multi-lumen tube is correctly positioned in both the stomach and the duodenum and for this reason many investigators prefer the separate placement of the gastric and duodenal tubes.

Steerable Burhenne-type catheters are available for rapid passage into the upper small intestine and can be used for jejunal biopsy, but they are expensive. The tip of these tubes can be manoeuvred by internal wires manipulated by proximal controls. Fluoroscopy is necessary.

Attachment of tubes to forceps in the biopsy channel of an upper digestive fibreoptic endoscopic by thread allows rapid visual placement. Alternatively, a guide wire can be positioned endoscopically and the diagnostic tube is then passed over it.

Intestine

Most operators construct their own tubes for intestinal work, but other tubes which have been used include the Miller-Abbot tube.

Scott-Harden tube

This useful tube is used by the radiologist for rapid intubation of the duodenum so that barium can be introduced into the small bowel. The tube consists of a gently curved stiff outer tube, which is positioned in the stomach so that the distal end rests at the level of the pylorus. An inner tube is then slid out and inserted through the pylorus. With experience this can be undertaken with great ease and rapidity. The procedure is superior to the use of internal stiffening wires.

Complications

Gastrointestinal intubation is free from complications when used for the short periods required to perform most diagnostic procedures. Minor pharyngeal irritation is about the only significant unpleasantness, but mucosal inflammation may occur. This interferes with endoscopy, which should, if required, be performed either first or after at least a week. If the tube remains in the stomach for more than a couple of days there is always the risk of gastric contents leaking past the gastro-oesophageal junction to cause oesophagitis and even stricture.

References

Hassan MA, Hobsley, M. Positioning of subject and nasogastric tube during a gastric secretion study. *Br Med J* 1970; i: 458–60

Hector RM. Improved technique of gastric aspiration. *Lancet* 1968; i: 15–6

Keller RT. A technique of intestinal intubation with the fibreoptic endoscope. *Gut* 1973; **14**: 143–4

Upper digestive endoscopy

The exact diagnosis of patients with haematemesis, dyspepsia and other upper abdominal symptoms cannot be made on the history alone. Diseases may simulate each other and different disorders can affect the same patient. Fibreoptic endoscopy with photography, biopsy and cytology has played a major role in evaluation and management. The technique is safe with a few contraindications, but requires training and experience to yield good results. It is usual for operators and assistants to wear disposable waterproof gloves. Special precautions are needed for patients known to carry hepatitis B virus, and those known or suspected of carrying HIV, including gowns and masks with visors. Endoscopy staff should be immunized against hepatitis B.

Instruments

There is a wide range of instruments from different manufacturers. For a panendoscopy a forward or oblique-viewing instrument is necessary (Figure 2). Some have a very large biopsy channel which allows the obtaining of especially satisfactory histology material. A modern standard instrument for routine use will be of about 11.5 mm external diameter and have a biopsy channel of 3.5 mm.

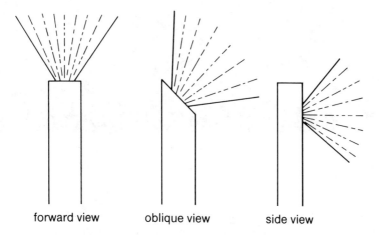

forward view   oblique view   side view

Figure 2 Viewing angles of endoscopes

For a full view of the lesser curve of the stomach, the duodenal bulb and the ampulla of Vater, a side-viewing instrument is sometimes necessary. This is the instrument usually employed for retrograde pancreatocholangiography.

There are available video endoscopy systems which display the image on a screen so that assistants may watch too. Alternatively a teaching side-piece can be attached to fibreoptic equipment, though with some loss of illumination.

Procedure (Figures 3 and 4)

To achieve good results the patient must be convinced of the value of the procedure. It should be explained that he will probably be awake (but drowsy) throughout and that with sedation he may have no recollection of the procedure.

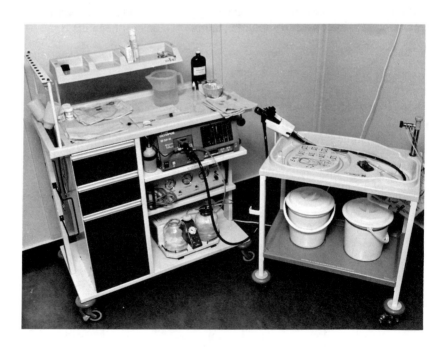

Figure 3 Equipment for upper digestive endoscopy

The stomach must be empty and this is achieved usually by fasting overnight, or for at least 4 hours. If the patient has had gastric suction for vomiting or if it is necessary to use some form of gastric intubation when brisk haematemesis or gastric outflow obstruction is present, it should be remembered that appearances of oesophageal, gastric lesser curve and antral erosions may be produced artefactually.

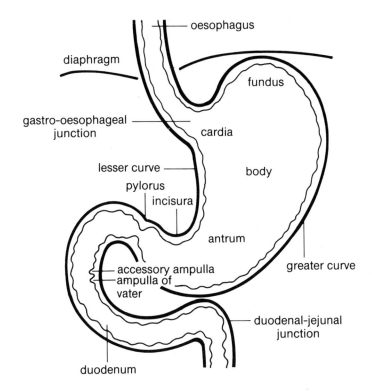

Figure 4 Diagram of upper gastrointestinal tract

False teeth should be removed. There is considerable variation in the techniques for preparation. A satisfactory one is to give atropine 0.6 mg and midazolam 5–10 mg intravenously immediately before the examination with the patient positioned on the left side. Smaller doses of midazolam (or none at all) may be required in patients with liver decompensation or respiratory failure. Larger or repeat doses may be required in the younger patient. It is rarely useful to exceed 2 mg midazolam and paradoxical hyperactivity can occur. The effect of benzodiazepine sedation can be rapidly reversed if necessary by flumazenil 500 mg intravenously. Doxapram 100 mg intravenously is less specific but can be useful too where excess respiratory depression occurs. A plastic gag with a central aperture to admit the endoscope is necessary to prevent the instrument being bitten by patients who have their own teeth. The endoscope is lubricated with water or clear jelly, and the light and suction equipment is tested before passage. The patient's head is flexed and the instrument tip is passed over the tongue to the oropharynx while an assistant holds the end with the controls. The patient is then asked to give a couple of swallows to assist passage into the oesophagus. If the patient does not comply the instrument may impact in the pharynx or enter the trachea. In either case the patient may choke and splutter, develop wheezing or coughing, and become cyanosed. If these occur the instrument should be withdrawn and a further attempt at passage made. If the trachea is entered the rough feel of the cartilages is experienced, and the branching pattern of the trachea is identified under direct vision. Guidance of the tip with a finger in the patient's mouth can be helpful.

In practice the oesophagus can usually be entered without difficulty.

Oesophagus

A good view of the oesophagus can be obtained on entry, but only usually over its lower two-thirds. Air insufflation assists vision, but should be used sparingly. The presence of macroscopic oesophagitis, Mallory–Weiss tears, stricture or carcinoma can be detected readily. Mallory–Weiss tears are produced by the effort of retching or vomiting. They are linear white ulcerated areas with surrounding erythema related to the level of the diaphragm. They usually occur at the gastro-oesophageal junction but in hiatus hernia are found in the cardia of the stomach. Oesophagitis is usually caused by retrograde reflux and extends proximally from the gastro-oesophageal junction. Mild oesophagitis is recognized by erythema, loss of surface glistening, vascular injection and friability. More severe changes lead to erosions, plaque formation and spontaneous bleeding. Discrete ulcers and benign strictures also occur, and in chronic oesophagitis the junction of the squamous and columnar epithelium can migrate proximally in Barrett's oesophagus.

Spiked forceps passed down the biopsy channel of the instrument can obtain multiple 2–3 mm samples to provide histological proof of diagnosis. It is best to take samples at least 5 cm above the gastro-oesophageal junction, since distal changes are common in healthy individuals. Samples are immediately immersed in formol saline. Cytology brushes can also be passed in the same way using a plastic catheter to protect the sample on withdrawal before immersing in fixative. It is recommended to take four biopsies and cytology brushings. If all are negative for carcinoma then this diagnosis is very unlikely in the oesophagus though this is less certain for the stomach. Occasionally a tight stricture cannot be passed, but in case of difficulty undue force must not be used. Gentle persuasion may pass the instrument through lesser strictures and give symptomatic relief. It may be possible to identify a hiatus hernia, though this is not always reliable.

The upper oesophagus and some of the pharynx can usually be seen with the narrow calibre instruments on withdrawal. Rigid oesophagoscopy by an ENT surgeon may be necessary if the postcricoid region is under suspicion.

Stomach

On passing over the normal gastro-oesophageal junction there is a change from pale pink mucosa to the orange-red mucosa of the stomach. This does not always correlate with histological change in epithelium. It is different from the high pressure zone of the lower oesophageal sphincter, and it normally lies below the level of the diaphragm, if this can be detected.

The greater curve and the antrum are easily viewed with air insufflation if necessary, but the rest of the stomach is more difficult to examine adequately. The greater curve is recognized by its rippling longitudinal folds; the antrum is smooth. The cardia can be seen well only by putting a J-bend on the end of the instrument when it reaches the pylorus and looking back towards the oesophagus. A partial view of the lesser curve is obtained as the instrument slides over it, but again a reverse loop may be necessary to view it completely. A sharp incisura may hide a small distal lesion. Often there is a pool of gastric juice on the greater curve; this may be aspirated, though care is needed to avoid damaging the mucosa. The pool can be removed by altering the patient's position slightly, or even by getting him to lie on his back temporarily so that a full view can be obtained.

Gastritis is often distal and is recognized by loss of surface glistening, granularity, vascular injection and friability. There may be haemorrhage or superficial erosions. Some gastritis is usual after gastric surgery, in which pyloric reflux is increased. Its significance is doubtful. Also transient erythema caused by retching is of no significance. In atrophic gastritis the stomach appears exceptionally smooth and often pale. In the autoimmune gastritis which causes pernicious anaemia an undulating knobbly appearance is characteristic. *Ulcers* are easily recognized; unless there has been recent bleeding they should ideally always have biopsies taken from the four quarters of the rim and from the base.

Carcinoma of the stomach can occur either as a malignant ulcer, sometimes with rolled undermined edges; or a polypoid lesion; or endoscopically normal: however, a small immobile stomach in which air is poorly retained should alert suspicion, and a mucosal biopsy may give a tissue diagnosis. A negative biopsy report never completely excludes a carcinoma, and if there is a clinical suspicion of malignancy then partial or total gastrectomy with excision biopsy should be considered.

The pylorus opens and closes during the examination. With a forward-viewing instrument it is usually easy to advance to the pylorus and wait for it to relax and allow entry. If the stomach is excessively mobile or if the stomach is an unusual shape the pylorus may be difficult to identify. It is best to withdraw the instrument further back into the body of the stomach and reorientate before proceeding. Free reflux of bile-stained fluid may be seen through the pylorus especially after cholecystectomy. It has no pathological significance but may foam and obscure the mucosa if air insufflation is used.

The pylorus is usually short, and of varying configuration as the peristaltic waves pass over. Ulcers can occur within the pyloric canal, and in the immediate pre- and post-pyloric regions, so that careful inspection in all stages of constriction and relaxation is rewarding. Uncommonly the pylorus is so tightly closed that the instrument cannot be passed further. If this is the case an injection of metoclopramide 10 mg intravenously relaxes muscular spasm. It also markedly increases duodenal mobility so that a further injection with atropine 0.6 mg, hyoscine 20 mg or glucagon 0.5 mg intravenously is necessary to view the duodenum.

Duodenum

Duodenal ulcers typically occur in the first part of the duodenal bulb, visible from the stomach before entering the pylorus. Thus inspection before entering is rewarding. The duodenal folds are circumferential and the mucosa is usually paler than the stomach. The view of the duodenal bulb is adequate, but the rest of the loop is often not seen well as the instrument is advanced, and a better view is obtained during withdrawal. The ampulla of Vater may be identifiable and can be located by the jets of bile which emerge from time to time. *Duodenitis*, with erythema, oedema and friability, may occur with or without ulcers. It can be patchy so a careful examination is necessary. Biopsy confirms doubtful appearances.

The area immediately distal to the pylorus is difficult to view properly with a forward-viewing instrument. An oblique-viewing instrument is often satisfactory but a side-viewing one is best. The pylorus is identified with a curve on the instrument so that the lens is facing forward. The instrument is then straightened and passed through the pylorus. The duodenum can be thoroughly inspected by rotating and advancing the instrument after abolishing muscle activity with atropine, hyoscine or glucagon. After passing the pylorus a rotation through 180° of the whole instrument brings the medial aspect of the duodenum into view. The accessory papilla can be seen and the more distal ampulla of Vater cannulated if desired.

Indications

(1) Investigation of dyspepsia, of abdominal pain and of iron deficiency anaemia.

(2) Diagnosis of haematemesis and melaena.
(3) Obtaining tissue samples for histology and cytology, especially in gastric ulcer, for microbiology in monilial oesophagitis, and in coeliac disease.
(4) Assessment of healing of peptic disease following medical treatment.
(5) Investigation of dyspepsia after gastric surgery.
(6) Evaluation of doubtful or negative barium meal appearances.
(7) Endoscopic retrograde cholangiopancreatography.
(8) Therapeutic endoscopy, dilation of strictures, injection of oesophageal varices and endoscopic papillotomy with retrieval of common bile duct stones. Oesophageal webs are disrupted by endoscopy, often without being visualized.
(9) Positioning diagnostic tubes by direct vision.
(10) Passage of ultrasound probes to investigate adjacent strictures.

ENDOSCOPIC RETROGRADE CHOLANGIOPANCREATOGRAPHY

Instruments

The instrument usually employed is the side-viewing duodenoscope, but the oblique and fine-calibre forward-viewing instruments have been used. A rotating lens system to give forward and lateral views is available but has not become popular. Both an image intensifier and facilities for taking radiographs are necessary.

Standard plastic catheters are suitable, though a finer tip is necessary for the accessory ampulla. Radiology is with 50 – 70% water-soluble iodine contrast medium.

Procedure

With the tip of the instrument in the second part of the duodenum the instrument is straightened by withdrawing the shaft after the ampulla has been identified. The catheter can then be advanced directly through the ampulla in the correct direction with the lens face-on to this structure.

The catheter tip is passed 1 – 2 cm into the duct and sufficient contrast injected under fluoroscopy to fill the main pancreatic duct and its major branches. Overfilling produces confusing radiographic appearances. The bile ducts may be demonstrated at the same time, but the anatomy of the ampulla is variable and it may be necessary to advance the catheter laterally to fill the pancreas, and then revise the position by withdrawal and advancing more rostrally to enter the bile ducts. These are then filled by further contrast injection and radiographic films are taken.

Pancreatic juice obtained at endoscopy can be examined for cells, and cytology may provide a tissue diagnosis.

Indications

(1) Confirmation of chronic pancreatitis and demonstration of potentially remediable strictures.
(2) Diagnosis of carcinoma of pancreas.
(3) Diagnosis of extrahepatic cholestasis where other methods have failed (prophylactic antibiotic cover is prudent).
(4) Identification and retrieval of common bile duct stones by papillotomy and basket or balloon extraction.

A success rate of 70–90% for cholangiography and 85–92% for pancreatography may be expected. The complication rate is 3.5–15%.

Relative contraindications

Recent acute pancreatitis and pancreatic pseudocyst.

Complications

(1) Ascending cholangitis.
(2) Acute pancreatitis (uncommon, although hyperamylasaemia is frequent).
(3) Haemorrhage after papillotomy.

CLEANSING

The fibreoptic endoscopes cannot be completely sterilized without damage. The best policy is to clean thoroughly between examinations and to submit them to antimicrobial treatment between lists.

Between examinations the lens and outer casings are wiped down with soap and water or chlorhexidine, followed by rinsing with water. A similar solution is sucked through the biopsy-suction channel, again followed by water.

Between endoscopy lists the whole instrument is immersed for 1 hour in activated glutaraldehyde with care to ensure filling of the biopsy channel. An alternative is to store the fibre bundle overnight in this solution. Low pressure ethylene oxide sterilization is a satisfactory method for treating the whole instrument.

PROPHYLAXIS OF SUB-ACUTE BACTERIAL ENDOCARDITIS

Though there is disappointingly little evidence that routine antibacterial prophylaxis has much influenced the prevalence of sub-acute bacterial endocarditis, it is recommended that patients with heart valve replacements or a prior history of sub-acute bacterial endocarditis receive antibacterial prophylaxis during endoscopy procedures. It is contentious whether it is useful to offer such treatment to all individuals with rheumatic heart disease.

For upper digestive endoscopy intravenous ampicillin 1 g given immediately prior to endoscopy is recommended. Where penicillin cannot be used alternatives include cefuroxime 750 mg, erythromycin 1 g (although this requires a large volume for intravenous use), and vancomycin 1 g (spectacularly expensive). For ERCP, colonoscopy and flexible sigmoidoscopy in patients at high risk, ampicillin 1 g plus gentamicin 80 mg, intravenously at the time of the procedure are recommended. Where penicillins cannot be used then gentamicin may be given alone.

Recommendations change from time to time as new information becomes available and new antibacterials are introduced.

References

Oi I. Fibre duodenoscopy and endoscopic pancreato-cholangiography. *Gastrointest Endosc* 1970; **17**: 59–62

Graham DY, Schwartz JT, Cain GC, Gyorkey F. Prospective evaluation of biopsy number in the diagnosis of oesophageal and gastric carcinoma. *Gastroenterology* 1982; **82**: 229–31

Shorvon P, Lees WR. Invasive ultrasound imaging. *Br J Hosp Med* 1985; May: 248–56

Gastrointestinal bleeding

Bleeding from the alimentary tract is an important manifestation of gastrointestinal disease. It may present as an unexplained anaemia, as the passage of black stool, as the passage of red blood per rectum, or by vomiting of fresh or altered blood.

The investigation of gastrointestinal bleeding involves answering two major questions: (1) is the patient still bleeding? and (2) where is the bleeding site?

Frank bleeding from the upper gastrointestinal tract, that is a site proximal to the duodenojejunal junction or ligament of Treitz, is usually obvious, presenting as a haematemesis or melaena stools. Fresh blood in the stools usually indicates rectal or colonic disease. However, it is possible for a bleeding lesion in the upper gastrointestinal tract to present with the passage of red blood per rectum; similarly a bleeding lesion in the caecum or ascending colon may cause melaena stools. The factors determining the degree of alteration of the blood in the gut include the site of the bleeding, the amount of blood lost and the motility of the bowel.

OCCULT BLOOD TESTS

Between 100 and 200 ml of blood in the gut is necessary to produce a tarry stool. With smaller volumes the stools are normally coloured and special tests are necessary to detect the presence of blood. Tests for occult blood are used either to detect the cause of an iron-deficiency anaemia or to help in the diagnosis of those lesions of the gut which are frequently associated with bleeding peptic ulcer, carcinoma and polyps. An average of 0.7 ml/day of blood is normally lost in the gastrointestinal tract.

The methods available to detect occult bleeding are chemical tests and the use of ^{51}Cr-labelled erythrocytes, the microscopic examination of the stool for erythrocytes, the microscopic demonstration of crystals of haemoglobin or its derivatives, and fluorimetric and spectroscopic tests for haemoglobin or its derivative porphyrins. Of these the most widely used are the chemical tests, although the radioactive method is the most accurate and reliable.

Chemical tests

Chemical tests are in universal use because of their simplicity, but it is extremely difficult to devise a standard chemical test which is neither too sensitive nor too insensitive.

Faecal samples for testing may be obtained from a stool sample, which is best taken from within a lump of faeces, from the material adhering to the sigmoidoscope or proctoscope, or from the faeces on the glove after rectal examination. It is possible by vigorous digital examination to cause sufficient trauma to the rectal mucosa to give a positive test for blood in the stool, so that a gentle examination is essential when procuring a sample of faeces for chemical examination.

There is a variety of commercial tests available. They are based on peroxidase-like activity in haemoglobin which causes the reagent used to develop a blue colour reaction. The most convenient sensitive test available is the guaiac test Hemachek, which is supplied as a kit so that the patient may send their own samples by post for examination. A specimen of stool is smeared on filter paper in a card. The reagent is added in the laboratory and a blue coloration indicates the presence of blood in the stool. This method reliably detects amounts of bleeding of 10 ml or more daily, and usually gives positive results if there is a loss of more than 2.5 ml daily. Haemoccult is a very much less sensitive guaiac test.

The Fecatwin system depends on two levels of sensitivity for guaiac testing, with additional confirmation of the presence of human haemoglobin by an immunological technique. It is rather too elaborate for routine use.

The benzidine test is no longer used because of the high incidence of cancer of the urinary bladder in persons concerned with its manufacture. Orthotolidine tests have become less popular with the development of the guaiac–haemoperoxidase tests, but laboratories can offer this test cheaply if immediate results are not essential.

False-positive reactions

The main objection to sensitive tests is the occurrence of false-positive reactions. These reactions are almost exclusively dietary in origin originating from the ingestion of red meat, uncooked vegetables, unboiled milk and fruit such as bananas. Opinions differ whether or not oral iron preparations can produce positive results, but it is probable that a weakly positive result may follow the ingestion of ferrous sulphate, ferrous fumarate and ferrous carbonate.

It must be stressed that negative occult blood tests do not exclude ulcerative or neoplastic lesions of the gastrointestinal tract.

The role of occult blood testing in *screening ostensibly healthy subjects* is controversial.

Where patients give a history consistent with *gastrointestinal bleeding* or are being investigated for iron-deficiency anaemia or suspected gastrointestinal disease a different approach is used.

(1)   Haemorrhoids, gingivitis and epistaxis are excluded.
(2)   Drugs, such as aspirin, which cause gastrointestinal bleeding are stopped.
(3)   Three separate stool samples are tested by routine methods.
(4)   If not all are positive then a ^{51}Cr-labelled erythrocyte study will yield further information; if this is not available then repeating the test after 3 days on a meat-free diet with only cooked vegetables (and taking bulk purgatives) may be helpful to exclude false positives.

In practice barium radiology and endoscopy are necessary in the diagnosis of difficult cases.

There is usually little doubt as to whether there is fresh blood in vomit. When altered blood or coloured material is present there may be uncertainty and the tests for occult blood mentioned above may be applied to the gastric aspirate or vomit. 'Coffee ground' vomit is not proven haematemesis until shown to contain blood in this way.

Test for dietary iron

Although the faecal occult blood tests should not give false-positive reactions there is sometimes difficulty in evaluating very dark stools. To exclude the presence of ingested iron as a complicating factor, a simple test may be helpful. This can also be used in testing for compliance with prescribed iron preparations and in detecting surreptitious self-medication.

Method

A small button of faecal material is emulsified in 2 mol/l hydrochloric acid and a drop of the emulsion is placed in the centre of a filter paper. After 1–2 minutes a thin, clear halo of fluid soaks into the paper around the drop. A drop of 2.5% potassium ferricyanide in aqueous solution is placed on the paper so that the haloes around the two drops meet at their periphery.

Interpretation

A positive result is the immediate appearance of a blue crescent at the interface between the two fluids. This indicates that there is iron in the stool and suggests that the patient is taking oral iron preparations. It is claimed that the test is not invalidated by blood in the stool.

^{99m}Technetium colloid test

When bleeding is brisk, then simply injecting ^{99m}Tc colloid intravenously and scanning the abdomen shortly afterwards can localize sites of haemorrhage.

Radiochromate-labelled erythrocytes

The measurement of gastrointestinal bleeding loss using ^{51}Cr-labelled red cells is the most reliable and the only quantitative test for gastrointestinal bleeding. ^{51}Chromium has proved a satisfactory label for red cells and hardly any is reabsorbed from the gut lumen. It is a gamma energy emitter.

Method

Twenty millilitres of blood are removed from the patient under investigation and the blood is transferred to a sterile universal container that has 5 ml acid citrate dextrose solution. The cells and plasma are separated. Between 100 and 300 mcCi sterile $Na_2^{51}CrO_4$ is added to the cells, mixed, and permitted to stand for 30 minutes at room temperature. At the end of incubation 50 mg ascorbic acid is added to reduce the free chromate to the non-tagging trivalent chromic salt. The cells are then washed two or three times in a mixture of the patient's plasma and physiological saline (3:100), resuspended in this mixture to a volume of about 25 ml and reinjected. Care is taken to prevent contamination of the patient's skin or bedclothes with the radioactive material as this could later affect the stool counts. The ^{51}Cr has a long half-life of 27.8 days and a patient can be studied for at least 4 weeks after the labelled erythrocytes have been reinjected.

A blood sample is taken after a suitable period of mixing, usually the fourth day, and further samples are taken during the period of the stool collection usually at 4–6 day intervals. Stools are collected over 24-hour periods into plastic bags or any other suitable container. The duration of stool collection varies according to the purpose of the test, but valid observations can be made later than 3 weeks after the initial labelling of the blood. The bags are weighed and the weight of the 24-hour stool output is obtained. The stool may either be dried or blended with a known volume of water. An alternative is for the collection to be bulked and counted whole. An aliquot is counted in a well-type scintillation counter. The blood content of a 24-hour faecal collection is then calculated using the formula:

$$\frac{\text{Total cpm in aliquot stool}}{\text{cpm/ml venous blood standard}} \times \frac{\text{Weight of 24-hour stool}}{\text{Weight of aliquot stool}}$$

Interpretation

The normal daily blood loss varies from 0.3–2.0 ml with an average of 0.7 ml. No dietary restrictions are necessary while the stools are collected, but the patient should be warned about the ingestion of salicylates and other potentially ulcerogenic drugs.

Having decided that the patient is bleeding from the gastrointestinal tract it is necessary to locate the bleeding site. A number of techniques may be employed, of which endoscopy is the most important.

OTHER TESTS

Radiology

The ability to obtain barium studies including a barium meal and follow-through, small bowel enema and a barium enema is essential in the investigation of gastrointestinal bleeding. Barium enemas should be by double-contrast technique unless there is a specific contraindication. There are also advantages in double-contrast barium meals, though they are not so readily available. The demonstration of a lesion does not prove that it is the bleeding site. This applies particularly to sigmoid diverticula. It is extremely difficult to decide upon the site of bleeding when two lesions are demonstrated, for example oesophageal varices and peptic ulcer. Portography may be performed when oesophageal and gastric varices are suspected. Arteriography is used to demonstrate lesions such as vascular anomalies, ulcers and neoplasia, and has been particularly recommended in the diagnosis of caecal tumours. Arteriography has also been used with success in the location of acute gastrointestinal haemorrhage by observing the site at which the dye leaks into the bowel lumen: it can be used to diagnose bleeding oesophageal varices.

Endoscopy

Upper digestive endoscopy, sigmoidoscopy and colonoscopy may all be required to determine the site of bleeding. Endoscopy is helpful because it may demonstrate that a lesion is actually bleeding. The performance of upper digestive endoscopy within 24 hours of admission with haematemesis greatly improves the diagnosis rate.

GASTROINTESTINAL BLEEDING IN LIVER DISEASE

If a patient is suspected to be bleeding from oesophageal varices, the sooner the correct diagnosis is made the more promptly appropriate therapy can be given. If varices are known to be present then the early use of terlipressin and a Sengstaken tube may be the best policy. However, it is preferable to obtain an urgent endoscopy since other lesions commonly bleed even in the patient with varices. Any blind intubation procedure may produce erosions or even Mallory-Weiss tears which can be mistakenly taken as the primary bleeding site at subsequent endoscopy.

References

Afifi AM *et al*. A simple test for ingested iron in hospital and domicilary practice. *Br Med J* 1966; i: 1021–2

Cameron AO. Gastro-intestinal blood loss measured by radioactive chromium. *Gut* 1960; **1**: 177–81

Irving JD. Northfield TC. Emergency arteriography in acute gastrointestinal bleeding. *Br Med J* 1976; ii: 929–31

Macrae FA, St John DJB, Caligiore P, Taylor LS, Legge JW. Optimal dietary conditions for Haemoccult testing. *Gastroenterology* 1982; 82: 899–903

Alavi A. Detection of gastrointestinal bleeding with ^{99m}Tc-sulfur colloid. *Semin Nucl Med* 1982; **12**: 126–38

CHAPTER 4

Oesophagus

The major symptoms of oesophageal disease are dysphagia, heartburn, postural dyspepsia and waterbrash. There are many tests of oesophageal function, though their interpretation depends on the definition of oesophageal disease.

OESOPHAGEAL ACID PERFUSION TEST

Pain of oesophageal origin may be identical to that of cardiac origin. The perfusion of 0.1 mol/l hydrochloric acid into the oesophagus is an easy and reasonably consistent way of reproducing the pain that arises from the gullet.

Method

The patient is seated in a highbacked chair and the oesophagus is intubated so that the distal end of the tube lies 30 cm from the teeth. Any convenient tube may be used. The position of the tube can be checked radiologically. The infusions to be used are suspended on a dripstand behind the patient who is unaware of which solution is being used and when the bottles are changed. Solutions of isotonic sodium chloride and 0.1 mol/l hydrochloric acid are made up in bottles and these are connected in turn to the oesophageal tube. Initially the isotonic sodium chloride is perfused at a rate of 10 ml/min for 10 min, followed by 20 ml/min for 5 min. Without the patient's knowledge the infusate is changed to 0.1 mol/l hydrochloric acid, initially 10 ml/min for 15 min followed by 20 ml/min for 15 min. If pain occurs the infusion is stopped and a solution of 0.05 mol/l sodium bicarbonate is infused. The perfusion can be repeated to confirm that a response is genuine. A standard twelve-lead electrocardiogram is obtained during any induced pain.

Interpretation

A *positive response* is pain produced by the acid but not by the saline solution. A positive test signifies pain of oesophageal origin but not necessarily oesophagitis. The test may be positive in normal subjects who have never suffered from pain and who have no evidence of oesophagitis. However, pain generally develops earlier (during the first 10 minutes of acid perfusion) in patients with oesophagitis. Patients with angina pectoris who have a positive response can usually distinguish the induced pain from that of angina pectoris.

A *negative test* is no pain being experienced during the perfusion but a negative response does not ensure that oesophageal disease is not the cause of the chest pain. Pain of similar severity induced both by saline and acid perfusion is also regarded as a negative test. Patients with angina pectoris usually have a negative response.

The procedure may induce an attack of angina pectoris (even with the infusion of saline) and then abnormalities of the electrocardiogram may be seen, but this is usually in patients with severe ischaemic heart disease.

This test is said to be a more reliable index of oesophageal origin for symptoms than endoscopy, but the two examinations are complementary. Some patients with a negative test respond with pain to infusion of foodstuffs which are suspected of causing symptoms.

References

Bernstein LM, Baker LA. Clinical test for oesophagitis. *Gastroenterology* 1958; **34**: 760–81
Winnan GR, Meyer CT, McCallum RW. Interpretation of the Bernstein test. A reappraisal of criteria. *Ann Intern Med* 1982; **96**: 320–2

OESOPHAGOSCOPY

Most of the disorders of the oesophagus affect the lower portion, which is conveniently inspected with a flexible fibreoptic panendoscope. If a patient has severe dysphagia a barium swallow examination is sometimes useful. The frequent co-existence of upper digestive abnormalities means that an oesophagogastroduodeno- scopy is an important investigation.

The upper oesophagus is often not well seen with the fibreoptic endoscope, and if a thorough examination of the post-cricoid region is required rigid oesophagoscopy under general anaesthetic is best. This technique also permits the taking of larger biopsy samples.

HISTOLOGY

At endoscopy it is important to take biopsies with forceps, and also to take cytology brushings if cancer is suspected.

The usefulness of histology in benign oesophagitis is more contentious.

The distal 2.5 cm usually has changes compatible with oesophagitis even in normal individuals, and it is not uncommon to find changes in health above this level. Probably the best site for biopsy is from 5–10 cm above the apparent gastro-oesophageal junction. The findings in oesophagitis include cellular infiltrates, increase in length of the dermal papillae and basal cell hyperplasia. Histology does not correlate well with symptoms, nor with macroscopic appearances at endoscopy.

References

Ismail-Beigi F, Pope CE. Distribution of the histological changes of gastroesophageal reflux in the distal oesophagus of man. *Gastroenterology* 1974; **66**: 1109–13

Ott DJ, Gelfand DW, Wu WC. Reflux oesophagitis: radiographic and endoscopic correlation. *Radiology* 1979; **130**: 583–8

Goldman H, Antonioli DA. Mucosal biopsy of the oesophagus, stomach and proximal duodenum. *Hum Pathol* 1982; **13**: 423–48

RADIOLOGY (Figures 5–9)

A variety of techniques has been described and each radiologist has his favourite, particularly when it comes to the diagnosis of hiatus hernia and gastro-oesophageal reflux.

The oesophagus should be examined both during and between swallows and in the upright and lying position. The patient is frequently tilted in the head-down position to demonstrate gastro-oesophageal reflux. When examining a patient for dysphagia the examination does not stop at failure to demonstrate an obstruction. Careful attention to oesophageal motility is essential. There are various manoeuvres to bring out diffuse oesophageal spasm, oesophageal rings and other motor disturbances of the oesophagus. The use of thick barium is one; even more informative is a 'bread bolus' in which a mouthful of bread is partially chewed and then swallowed with a mouthful of barium solution. The patient must report any pain or discomfort during the act of swallowing and at such time particular attention is paid to oesophageal contractions.

Cineradiology is of great value and has the advantage that both the radiologist and the clinician together can review and discuss the motility and function of the oesophagus at some time after the radiological examination.

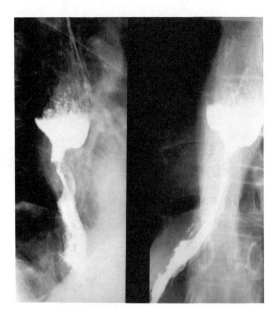

Figure 5 Barium swallow. Typical 'shouldering' due to a carcinoma of the lower two-thirds of the oesophagus

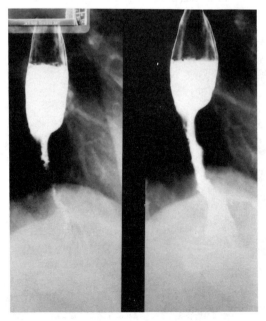

Figure 6(a) Barium swallow showing carcinoma of the lower two-thirds of the oesophagus

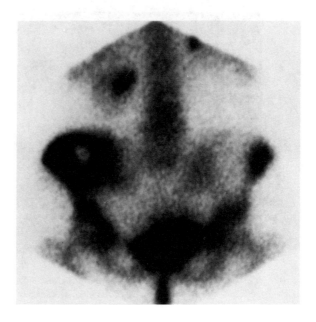

Figure 6(b) ^{99m}Technecium isotope bone scan showing destruction of bone by metastasis

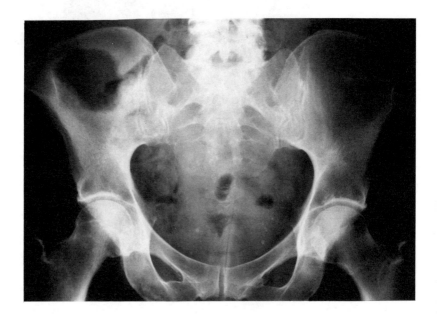

Figure 6(c) Radiograph of the pelvis showing a 'hole' in the right iliac bone due to metastases

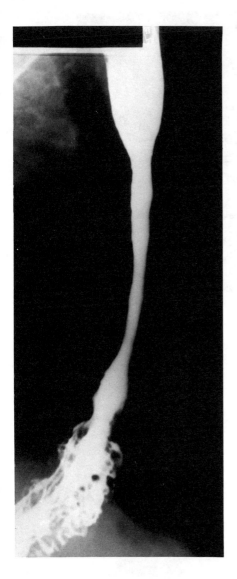

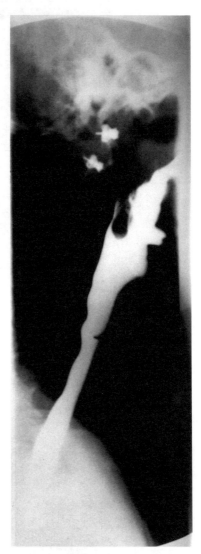

Figure 7 Barium swallow showing a long
peptic stricture

Figure 7 Barium swallow showing an
oesophageal web

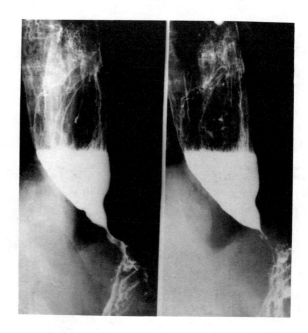

Figure 9(a) Barium meal showing achalasia of oesophagus

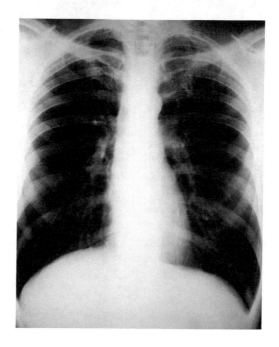

Figure 9(b) Chest radiograph showing no air in the fundus of the stomach

MANOMETRY

Pressure recording from the oesophagus is increasingly being used in clinical medicine. Oesophageal motility studies are particularly valuable in the early diagnosis of achalasia of the cardia and in various motor disorders. The apparatus consists of a multichannel pressure recorder and a series of tubes to conduct the oesophageal pressure. Scrupulous attention to detail is necessary to obtain interpretable results.

Method

Intraluminal pressures can be recorded either by water-filled polyethylene tubes with lateral orifices or by balloon-tipped tubes. Sphincter pressures registered by the latter method are usually greater than with the open tubes. Three tubes are sealed together and the lateral orifices, or balloons, are set at 5 cm intervals so that simultaneous recordings can be made from three sites. Pressure changes are transmitted via transducers to a multichannel direct recorder (any recorder used for cardiopulmonary studies can be used). Swallowing and respiratory movements are recorded. Pressure recordings are taken in the stomach, at the gastro-oesophageal region and in the oesophagus the both during and between swallowing. The patient can be studied while drinking 10 ml of water or during a 'dry' swallow. Recordings are made with the tube fixed at different levels throughout the oesophagus ('station' method). There is controversy over whether a rapid pull-through technique is superior; it certainly gives different results from the standard station method.

Ambulatory 24-hour manometry is described but not yet standard practice.

Interpretation

Normal swallowing

On withdrawal of the tube from stomach to oesophagus there is a pressure reversal, the positive intra-abdominal pressure changing to a negative intrathoracic pressure. The normal resting intra-oesophageal pressure is between $+2$ and -20 cm water. When the patient swallows, a positive peristaltic wave of $40-80$ cm water, which is co-ordinated and regular, sweeps down the oesophagus. A zone of increased pressure is present $2-3$ cm above the gastro-oesophageal junction. This relaxes during swallowing, the relaxation preceding the arrival of the peristaltic wave.

Achalasia of the cardia

There is an absence of regular peristaltic contractions in the body of the oesophagus and there is failure of the lower oesophageal sphincter to relax during swallowing. The resting tone of the lower oesophageal sphincter is normal.

Diffuse spasm

Inco-ordinate (tertiary) contractions of the lower half to one-third of the oesophagus will be recorded and the resting pressure in the oesophagus may be raised to 200–400 cm water. The lower oesophageal sphincter functions normally although it may be included in the inco-ordinate contractions.

Scleroderma

The lower three-quarters of the oesophagus shows feeble simultaneous contractions while the upper quarter retains normal function. There is a decline in the tone of the sphincter. At a later stage the motility disorder resembles achalasia of the cardia.

Hiatus hernia

Four characteristic changes have been described.

(1)   A double respiratory reversal point on withdrawing the recording device through the hernial sac: that is positive pressure in the stomach, negative in the hiatus, positive in the hernial sac and finally negative as the sphincter is passed.
(2)   Two pressure peaks representing the oesophageal hiatus and the gastro-oesophageal sphincter.
(3)   A plateau of positive pressure in the hernia.
(4)   An increased length of the zone of high pressure.

Symptoms of oesophageal reflux are sometimes but not always associated with hiatus hernia.

References

Goodall RJR, Hay DJ, Temple JG. Assessment of the rapid pull-through technique in oesophageal manometry. *Gut* 1980; **21**: 169–73

Arndorfer RC, Stef JF, Dodds WJ, Lineman JH, Hogan WJ. Improved infusion system for intraluminal oesophageal manometry. *Gastroenterology.* 1977; **73**: 23–7

Clark J, Moossa AR, Skinner DB. Pitfalls in the performance and interpretation of oesophageal function tests. *Surg Clin North Am* 1976; **66**: 20–37

REFLUX STUDIES

The failure of other tests to discriminate absolutely between normals and patients thought to have oesophageal reflux symptoms has led to more elaborate procedures.

Method

Short-term studies

Intra-oesophageal pH is measured by an electrode or radio-pill. The probe is positioned in the stomach and then withdrawn up the oesophagus past the high-pressure zone (as defined by manometry) with continuous pH monitoring. The test is repeated after instillation of 250–300 ml 0.1 mol/l HCl in the stomach, and with both tests the level at which the pH reaches 4 is recorded. In a positive test pH falls below 4 above the high-pressure zone. A further modication is to position the pH electrode 5 cm above the high-pressure zone and perform manoeuvres such as head tilting, deep breathing, Valsalva and coughing to precipitate reflux as defined by a fall in pH of 2 units or more.

Long-term studies

The pH electrode is positioned 5 cm proximal to the high-pressure zone and taped into position. Radiographic screening before and after the test confirms that there is no displacement. Continuous monitoring is then conducted for 24 hours. Any fall in pH of 2 units or more which lasts 1 minute or more is recorded as a reflux episode. The number and duration of reflux episodes is recorded. The length of time oesophageal pH is below 4 is the best discriminant and should be less than 6% time supine and 10.5% time erect in normals.

A further technique is that of gastro-oesophageal scintiscanning after ingestion of a meal labelled with [99m]technetium colloid. This has not yet been fully evaluated and the method described has the disadvantage of still requiring intubation.

References

Stanciu C, Hoare RC, Bennett JR. Correlation between manometric and pH tests for gastro-oesophageal reflux. *Gut* 1977; **18**: 536-40

Fisher RS, Malmud IS, Roberts GS, Lobis IF. Gastroesophageal scintiscanning to detect and quantitate reflux. *Gasteroenterology* 1976; **70**: 301-8

Branicki FJ, Evans DF, Ogilvie AL, Atkinson M, Hardcastle JD. Ambulatory monitoring of oesophageal pH in reflux oesophagitis using a portable radio-telemetry capsule. *Gut* 1982; **23**: 992-8

Emde C, Garner A, Blum AL. Technical aspects of intraluminal pH-metry in man: Current status and recommendations. *Gut* 1987; **28**: 1177-88

Johnsson F, Joelsson B, Isberg P-E. Ambulatory 24-hour intraoesophageal monitoring in the diagnosis of gastrooesophageal reflux disease. *Gut* 1987; **28**: 1145-50

Schindbleck NE, Heinrich C, König A, Dendorfer A, Pace F, Müller-Lissner SA. Optimal thresholds, sensitivity and specificity of long-term pH-metry for the detection of gastro-oesophageal reflux disease. *Gastroenterology* 1987; **93**: 85-90

Johnsson F, Joelsson B. Reproducibility of ambulatory oesophageal pH monitoring. *Gut* 1988; **29**: 886-9

ISOTOPE SWALLOW

Method

While lying under a gamma camera the fasting patient is asked to swallow a small volume of water containing 100-300 microcuries of ^{99m}technetium colloid. This is conveniently injected into the mouth by a short flexible tube connected to a 20 ml syringe. The isotope can be followed into the stomach, and normally at least 90% of the activity should have left the oesophagus in 15 seconds. Healthy young subjects generally clear all the activity into the stomach within 10 seconds. The test is repeated twice to ensure reproducibility. The test may be extended by then allowing the patient to sit up and swallow 300 ml 0.1 mol/l HCl flavoured with orange juice. Distal oesophageal scanning is then repeated with the patient supine to see if spontaneous reflux occurs from the stomach. If no spontaneous reflux is seen then external abdominal pressure can be applied with a thigh blood-pressure cuff inflated to 20, 40, 60, 80 and finally 100 mmHg external pressure at half-minute intervals, with continuous oesophageal scanning.

Interpretation

Normally 10% or less of the isotope remains in the oesophagus at 15 seconds, and clearance is smoothly progressive. At least two out of three swallows should be abnormal before the test is regarded as positive. No reflux within the oesophagus or from the stomach should be seen.

In achalasia the pattern is grossly distorted with accumulation of isotope in an akinetic oesophagus.

In oesophageal dysmotility clearance is delayed and incomplete during the examination. There may be oscillation of bolus of isotope, indicating intra-oesophageal reflux.

In gastro-oesophageal reflux isotope re-enters the oesophagus from the stomach. This test is most helpful when the reflux is spontaneous rather than when it has to be induced by raising abdominal pressure artificially. In children significant reflux is often gross, and a simple ultrasonography technique may be preferable.

Precaution

Secondary motility disorders are common, and an upper digestive endoscopy is obligatory to the interpretation of isotope swallow results. Not only may oesophageal strictures or carcinomas affect motility, but also apparently separate problems such as a duodenal ulcer can do so too. The presence of isotope in a large hiatus hernia may masquerade either as delayed emptying or as gastro-oesophageal reflux: the pattern can be recognised for what it is with experience.

The most serious drawbacks of isotope studies are that motility disorders are common with advancing age and may be not explain symptoms, and that a separate classification of disease is required from those used in endoscopy, histology and manometry.

Despite these problems isotope swallow studies are very useful since they are convenient, quick and cheap.

References

Kaul B, Petersen H, Grette K, Erichsen H, Myrvold HE. Scintigraphy, pH measurement, and radiology in the evaluation of gastro-oesophageal reflux. *Scand J Gastroenterol* 1985; **20**: 289–94

Kaul B, Petersen H, Grette K, Myrvold HE. Reproducibility of gastro-oesophageal reflux scintigraphy and the standard acid reflux test. *Scand J Gastroenterol* 1986; **21**: 795–8

Velasco N, Pope CE, Gannan RM, Roberts P, Hills LD. Measurement of esophageal reflux by scintigraphy. *Dig Dis Sci* 1984; **29**: 977–82

De Caestecker JS, Blackwell JN, Adam RD, Hannan WJ, Brown J, Heading RC. Clinical value of radionuclide oesophageal transit measurement. *Gut* 1986; **27**: 659–66

Nail DR, Moore DJ. Ultrasound diagnosis of gastro-oesophageal reflux. *Arch Dis Child* 1984: **59**: 366–7

Stomach

GASTRIC EMPTYING

Isotope tests

A normal meal can be labelled with ^{99m}technetium, e.g. as ^{99m}Tc-diethylene-triamine-pentacetic acid (DTPA). The supine patient is scanned half-hourly after this has been consumed, till activity has left the stomach. Emptying is exponential, so the half-life of meals in the stomach is a useful measurement. This is normally 60–90 min, compared with 40–60 min in uncomplicated duodenal ulcers and 75–100+ min in duodenal ulcers with gastric outflow obstruction.

More sophisticated techniques have been described, such as labelling the solid phase of a meal (chicken liver) with ^{99m}technetium and simultaneously labelling the liquid phase with ^{113m}indium. However, no system is foolproof since isotope labels can separate from solids, and the size and physical state of particles may change during the procedure.

Radiology

The time taken for a barium meal to clear the stomach is normally 2–3 hours. Prolongation of this time may indicate disease, but is an unphysiological test. Gastric barium will complicate any early surgery for obstruction. Solid radio-opaque markers can be used, e.g. 10 mm lengths of 16F nasogastric tube, which should mostly clear the stomach in 4 hours and almost all have left in 6 hours.

Ultrasonography

Serial real-time scans parallel to the long axis of the stomach or of the antrum can be used to calculate gastric emptying of physiological meals. This is a useful completely non-invasive test, though probably unnecessary in children with pyloric stenosis where physical examination and observation confirm the diagnosis. The presence of gastric air often prevents accurate assessment.

Dye dilution

This requires nasogastric intubation. A test meal of 750 ml of water is drunk, and either before or after ingestion phenol red 30 ppm is added. After thorough mixing a 7–8 ml aliquot is withdrawn and 20 ml phenol red 500 ppm is added. After further thorough mixing a second aliquot is withdrawn, and from the concentrations gastric volume can be calculated. The procedure is repeated at intervals to determine the rate of reduction of gastric volume. In normal subjects the half-life of gastric volume is 11 min, and the emptying time is 22 min.

References

Chaudhuri TK. Use of ^{99m}DTPA for measuring gastric emptying time. *J Nucl Med* 1974; **15**: 391–5

Heading RC, Tothill P, McLoughlin GP, Shearman DJC. Gastric emptying rate measurement in man. *Gastroenterology* 1976; **71**: 45–50

Collins PJ, Horowitz M, Cook DJ, Harding PE, Shearman DJC. Gastric emptying in normal subjects. *Gut* 1983; **24**: 1117–25

Fieldman M, Smith HJ, Simon TR. Gastric emptying of solid radiopaque markers. *Gastroenterology* 1984; **87**: 895–902

Bateman DN, Whittingham TA. Measurement of gastric emptying by real-time ultrasonography. *Gut* 1982; **23**: 524–7

Bolondi L, Bortolotti M, Santi V, Calletti T, Gaiana S, Labo G. Measurement of gastric emptying time by real-time ultrasonography. *Gastroenterology* 1985; **89**: 752–9

Holt S, Cervantes J, Wilkinson AA, Wallace JHK. Measurement of gastric emptying rate in humans by real-time ultrasonography. *Gastroenterology* 1986; **90**: 918–23

George JD. New clinical method for measuring gastric emptying: the double sampling test method. *Gut* 1968; **9**: 237–42

Hunt JN. A modification of the method of George for studying gastric emptying. *Gut* 1974; **15**: 812–3

Hurwitz A. Measuring gastric volumes by dye dilution. *Gut* 1981; **22**: 85–93

GASTRIC ACID SECRETION

The estimated output of acid is a widely used test of gastric function. Various stimulants have been used in the past, but they have been largely superseded by the introduction of *pentagastrin*. This is a pentapeptide containing the key C-terminal sequence of gastrin, i.e. tryptophane-methionine-asparagine-phenylalanine-NH$_2$.

There are many different techniques, but as long as a department performs the test in a standard way the results will be similar. Results are poor when the test is performed by the most junior nurse in the course of other routine ward duties, and ideally each hospital should have a small number of specially trained nurses or technicians to undertake these tests.

Short pentagastrin test

Method

Antacids are stopped at least a day before the test. Ideally atropinics, tricyclic antidepressants, H_2-receptor antagonists or omeprazole should be discontinued a week before the test. The patient is weighed. After an overnight fast a nasogastric tube is passed into the stomach. The patient is positioned on the left side and the aspiration ports are positioned under the surface of the pool of gastric juice by one of the methods detailed in Chapter 1. Occasionally fluoroscopy or a radiographic film are necessary to locate the tube, but in the hands of an experienced operator this is not generally required. The patient is asked to spit out saliva during the test. The stomach is aspirated and the overnight secretion is discarded.

Pentagastrin 6 mcg/kg is then given subcutaneously (or intramuscularly). In the 10 minutes after the injection, the gastric secretion is collected either by intermittent syringe aspiration or by electric suction pump with a sub-atmospheric pressure of 5 mmHg. This collection is discarded. All the gastric secretion from 10–30 minutes after the pentagastrin injection is collected and saved. The volume and pH are measured and titratable acidity is measured by titration against 0.01 mol/l NaOH to pH 7. The tube is removed and the whole test usually complete within 45 minutes.

The test described above is based on the knowledge that 6 mcg/kg pentagastrin is a maximal stimulus when given either subcutaneously, intramuscularly, or intravenously as a bolus or infusion, and that the maximal effect is almost always seen 10–30 minutes after injection. However, after gastric surgery the maximal response may not be seen until 12 mcg/kg pentagastrin is given. It is preferable to compare tests before and at a fixed interval after gastric surgery, and in this case it is best to use 6 mcg/kg for both.

Results

pH. This is the logarithmic measurement of the hydrogen ion content. In a normal stomach pH is 1–3 units, and in achlorhydria it is 7–8 units.

Volume. Volume is low (or secretion absent) in hypochlorhydria. It is high in duodenal ulcer and very high in gastric hypersecretion secondary to gastrinoma.

Titratable acidity. Using 1 ml of specimen, the volume of 0.01 mol/l NaOH used to titrate to pH 7 as measured by the pH meter is equivalent to 100x the mmol hydrogen ion present. This is multiplied by volume to give titrable acidity per 20 minute sample, and by three to give a peak acid output (PAO) in mmol/hour.

Interpretation

There is a large individual variation in tests and a large overlap between groups with different conditions. Results will depend on patients' build, and height and lean body mass are both important. For adults these are usually neglected, but in children results should be expressed as mcmol/kg/hour.

Men secrete more gastric acid than women, and secretion falls off with advancing age. Race is also a factor, but the data are conflicting. To assist understanding, Table 1 shows the results of the test outlined above during 1 year in patients in Dundee who also had a full upper digestive endoscopy within 6 weeks.

Table 1 Short pentagastrin test: PAO (mmol/hour)

	Men				Women		
	n	Mean	Range		n	Mean	Range
Normal	41	30	0.6 – 56.6		26	20	0 – 45.6
Duodenal ulcer (no duodenitis)	61	42**	21.7 – 72.9		38	35***	6.6 – 52.2
Duodenitis (no duodenal ulcer)	63	36*	0 – 84.8		18	28**	12.5 – 51.1
Oesophagitis	77	34*	1.6 – 84.8		50	28**	1 – 52.2
Gastritis and gastric erosions	63	33	2.4 – 84.8		36	28**	1 – 51.1
Pyloric and prepyloric ulcer	23	33	9.9 – 60.2		15	26	0 – 39.7
Benign gastric ulcer	10	29	1.6 – 41.9		12	19	10 – 35.7
Any type vagotomy and/or drainage (no gastrectomy)	47	26	0.1 – 47.7		22	19	0 – 35.7

*$p < 0.05$;   **$p < 0.01$;   ***$p < 0.001$
Differences calculated versus normal endoscopy

The distribution of values is not parametric. However, for an individual the results are highly reproducible, with a coefficient of variation of 4.6%.

Normal acid secretion is usually taken to be 10–30 mmol/hour for women and 15–40 mmol/hour for men. Studies of endoscopy-normal dyspeptic patients and apparently healthy volunteers show that values often fall outside these ranges. Younger subjects have rather higher values, and over the age of 50 years the difference between the sexes becomes less marked. Any disease apart from *pernicious anaemia* may be found in the presence of normal acid secretion.

Benign gastric ulcer is in general associated with normal acid secretion. However, the more proximal the ulcer the lower the acid output; conversely, patients with pyloric and pre-pyloric ulcers tend to be hypersecretors.

Achlorhydria. The absence of any titrable acid in a stomach whose contents have a pH of 6 or more after an adequate pentagastrin test in a patient who has not had a gastric resection of cholecystectomy is undoubtedly achlorhydria. If these conditions are not met the definition becomes arbitrary and the expression should not be used.

Achlorhydria may occur in apparently normal individuals and becomes commoner with ageing. It is also found in the autoimmune gastritis of pernicious anaemia, in iron deficiency, in atrophic gastritis and in 18% of cases of gastric cancer. Benign peptic ulcer very rarely occurs in achlorhydria.

Reduced acid secretion. A PAO of less than 10 mmol/hour in women and less than 15 mmol/hour in men virtually excludes active duodenal ulcer. This may be important where radiology shows only deformity of the duodenal cap and endoscopy does not identify an active ulcer in a patient with dyspepsia. A low acid output is characteristic of gastric cancer, but is certainly not pathognomonic and is not always associated with the condition.

Increased acid secretion is characteristically found in duodenal ulcer, though half of these patients have a normal acid output. It is occasionally caused by gastrinoma or hypercalcaemia. The hypersecretion tends to be more marked in patients with duodenal ulcer complications.

Basal acid secretion

This yields variable results and does not add to the diagnostic usefulness of the PAO where duodenal ulcer is suspected. The test should only be performed in special circumstances, e.g. when gastrinoma is suspected.

Method

The patient is intubated after an overnight fast. The overnight juice is aspirated and its volume, pH and titratable acidity are measured. The stomach is then aspirated for 1 hour without any stimulation and the volume, pH and titratable acidity are measured. To ensure the most reliable results the collection should be fractionated into 4 x 15 min periods and the results of the analyses summated. The coefficient of variation between fractions is about 50%, but at least it provides some indication that the test is adequately performed. The basal acid output (BAO) is expressed in mmol/hour. Pentagastrin-stimulated PAO should then usually be measured to obtain the maximum useful information.

Results

In *achlorhydria* the BAO and the PAO are both nil, and the PAO is much more reliable. In duodenal ulcer the BAO is raised, as is the acidity and volume of overnight juice: the ratio of BAO/PAO is the same as in normals.

In *gastro-induced hypersecretion*, e.g. with a gastrinoma, the BAO is at least 60% of the PAO, and the two values are usually the same. The PAO may not be markedly raised.

Acid output after surgery

Measurement of gastric acid output after gastric surgery is important in the assessment of symptoms and of the adequacy of the surgeon's attempts to reduce acid secretion. Surgery often interferes with the test: collection of gastric juice is almost inevitably incomplete after a partial gastrectomy and may also be incomplete after a pyloroplasty. The results must therefore be treated with caution. In addition the acid output is lower in the early postoperative period than that observed 6–12 months later. A standard regimen of performing the test at a fixed interval after operation should be employed. One approach is to measure acid output on the 7–10th day immediately before discharge. Another is to recall all patients 6 months after surgery, but unfortunately at this time the asymptomatic patients are often reluctant to undergo further tests.

Insulin test

This test, devised by Hollander, remains popular with doctors despite the disadvantages to the patients who usually experience unpleasant symptoms. It has to be supervised with great care and regrettably, as with the older augmented histamine test, deaths have occurred.

Method

After an overnight fast a nasogastric tube is passed. An injection of 50 ml of 50% glucose is drawn up into a syringe. The basal acid output is measured. An intravenous cannula is inserted into a peripheral vein. 0.2 units/kg of soluble insulin are injected intravenously, and 8 x 15 min fractional collections of gastric juice are made over 2 hours. Blood is taken for laboratory measurement of glucose at 30 min intervals; an adequate test requires the absence of significant increase in gastric secretion in the presence of a blood glucose fall to 1.7 mmol/l or less.

Patients usually feel unwell during the test, and if symptoms are severe or unconsciousness occurs the test must be terminated by the injection of glucose.

Interpretation

Not the least of the problems with this test is the lack of agreement about how to interpret it. Two criteria are:

(1)   *Hollander's criteria for incompleteness of vagotomy*
       Either increase in titratable acidity of 20 mmol/l over BAO in two successive 15 min periods, *or* an acidity in any sample of 10 mmol/l if there is no titratable acidity in the basal sample.

(2)   *Glasgow criterion for incompleteness of vagotomy*
       An increase in acid output of three times the BAO in any sample. The basal output is conveniently taken as the mean acidity of the 4 x 15 min basal periods, which may be directly compared with each of the 8 x 15 min periods after insulin.

2-Deoxy-D-glucose test

This analogue of glucose causes vagal stimulation, possibly by interfering with the metabolism of glucose by the central nervous system. The 2-deoxy-D-glucose is infused intravenously over 10 minutes in a dose of 40–70 mg/kg body weight. After the infusion there is a rise in blood sugar despite which the patient may experience the symptoms of hypoglycaemia. There is a prompt rise in gastric acid output in the presence of an intact vagus; a complete vagotomy is indicated by no acid response.

Despite theoretical attractions of greater potency it has proved toxic in use and probably confers no advantage over the insulin test.

Similarly the intravenous injection of tolbutamide 1 g reduces blood glucose, but it is no better than insulin for this purpose.

Pre- and postoperative pentagastrin stimulation

Kronborg showed that the comparison of augmented histamine tests before and after surgery gave as good results as the insulin test in predicting recurrence of peptic ulceration. The pentagastrin test is both shorter and safer and it should yield similar results to the augmented histamine test. This is an attractive technique as most patients will have a measurement of gastric acid output before surgery.

Interpretation

The average reduction of PAO in a successful vagotomy is 60–70%. A postoperative PAO greater than 50% of preoperative PAO suggests incomplete vagotomy, and if the two values are the same the attempt at vagotomy can be regarded as having definitely failed.

If the PAO 10 days after surgery is >20 mmol/hour in men or >18 mmol/hour in women the risk of recurrent ulcer is about 25%.

Indications for gastric acid studies

(1) *Diagnosis of pernicious anaemia.* Achlorhydria is obligatory, and PAO is nil. The test is not often used now because there are other direct means of diagnosing pernicious anaemia.

(2) *Diagnosis of hypersecretion secondary to hypergastrinaemia* as in gastrinoma (Zollinger–Ellison syndrome). G-cell hyperplasia, retained antrum after gastric surgery, hypercalcaemia and short bowel syndrome. The basal hour volume is usually > 200 ml, BAO > 15 mmol/hour, BAO/PAO > 60% and PAO usually > 50 mmol/hour.

(3) *Pre- and postoperatively in peptic ulcer surgery.* Most gastroenterologists believe that the measurement of gastric secretion should neither influence the decision when to operate nor determine the type of operation. A record of the change in acid output with surgery is a useful measure of the completeness of the vagotomy and the risk of recurrence.

(4)   *Assessement of response to H$_2$-receptor antagonist treatment*. The dose of drugs in an unresponsive duodenal ulcer and in hypergastrinaemia-induced hypersecretion can be titrated to reduce PAO to subnormal levels.

(5)   *Selection of operation for oesophageal reflux*. It has been claimed that hypersecretors with oesophagitis do well after vagotomy, without the need for major plastic procedures to the cardia.

(6)   Occasionally in the *differentiation of benign from malignant gastric ulcer*. If a gastric ulcer exists in the presence of achlorhydria it should be regarded as malignant. In practice the PAO is of little help in management because all gastric ulcers should have a biopsy taken at the time of gastroscopy.

Alternative techniques – sham feeding test for gastric secretion

Acid secretion may be stimulated by the technique of sham-feeding, where food is chewed and then spat out without swallowing any. Though attractively simple and harmless, the procedure is unaesthetic and has not gained wide popularity. The concept of testing gastric pH intra-operatively during pentagastrin infusion to ensure completeness of vagotomy has appeal but prolongs time in theatre and increases the morbidity.

References

Kronborg O, Anderson D. Acid response to sham-feeding as a test for completeness of vagotomy. *Scand J Gastroenterol* 1980; **15**: 119–21

Fieldman M, Richardson CT, Fordtran JS. Experience with sham-feeding as a test for vagotomy. *Gastroenterology* 1980; **79**: 792–5

Radiotelemetry

A more modern method is the use of the radiotelemeter capsule. This is 10 x 25 mm and contains a glass pH electrode, transistor oscillator and replaceable mercury battery in a polyacrylate body. The capsule is swallowed and located in the body by positioning the receiving aerial on the skin over the maximal signal. The gastric pH can be measured directly, and if desired a complete pH profile of the gut obtained before recovery from the faeces.

Intravenous [99m]technetium

Another approach is the intravenous injection of 1 mCi [99m]technetium 15 min after pentagastrin 6 mcg/kg subcutaneously. A scintiscan over the stomach is performed 15 min later and the activity is directly proportional to acid output ($r = 0.87$). This technique may also be useful for the identification of ectopic gastric tissue in a Meckel's diverticulum.

Serum gastrin

There is a whole family of circulating gastrins but modern assays concentrate on G17. This is the 'small' gastrin with 17 amino acid residues and including one sulphated tyrosine residue. Levels rise in the circulating blood in response to a meal.

Interpretation

The normal range in fasting serum is 5–50 pmol/l (1 pmol/l is the equivalent of 2.1 pg/ml). It is not raised in duodenal ulcer disease and is of no help in diagnosis unless a gastrinoma or G-cell hyperplasia is suspected because of severe, atypical or recurrent ulceration. The diagnosis then rests on a BAO/PAO ratio > 60% and a fasting serum gastrin of > 100 pmol/l.

Problems of interpretation

(1) The serum gastrin may be elevated without gastric hypersecretion in pernicious anaemia, hypochlorhydria, rheumatoid arthritis and in renal failure.
(2) The serum gastrin is low when gastric surgery removes the antrum, but rises when vagotomy is performed with antral retention. Often postvagotomy values are three to four times the upper limit of normal in the absence of hypersecretion.
(3) In gastrinoma the serum gastrin may be below 100 pmol/l. If the diagnosis is suspected, fasting blood is taken for gastrin assay followed by an injection of secretin 1–2 u/kg. Gastrin is measured in a blood sample taken 5 min later, and a rise in levels of > 50% is positive.

Serum pepsinogen

This can be measured enzymatically or by radioimmunoassay (RIA). The Group I pepsinogens have an upper limit of normal measured enzymatically of 50 units/ml, and by RIA of 100 mcg/ml. They do not vary through the day, and correlate fairly well with PAO ($r=0.74$). Pepsinogen is elevated in renal failure, which may not be associated with gastric hypersecretion.

References

Baron JH. *Clinical Tests of Gastric Secretion: history, methodology and interpretation.* London: MacMillan 1978

Taylor TV, Holt S, McLoughlin GR, Heading RC. A single scan technique for estimating acid output. *Gastroenterology* 1979; **77**: 1241 – 4

Turner MD, Tuxill JL, Miller LL, Segal HL. Measurement of pepsin I (gastricsin) in human gastric juice. *Gastroenterology* 1967; **53**: 905 – 11

Ardeman S, Chanarin I. A method for the assay of human gastric intrinsic factor and for the detection and titration of antibodies against intrinsic factor. *Lancet* 1963; ii: 1350 – 4

Johnston D, Jepson K. Use of pentagastrin in a test of gastric acid secretion. *Lancet* 1967; ii: 585 – 8

Hollander F. The insulin test for the presence of intact nerve fibres after vagal operations for peptic ulcer. *Gastroenterology* 1946; **7**: 607 – 14

Gillespie G, Elder JB, Smith IS, Kennedy F, Gillespie IE, Kay AW, Campbell EHG. Analysis of basal acid secretion and its relation to the insulin response in normal and duodenal ulcer patients. *Gastroenterology* 1972; **62**: 903 – 11

Kronborg O. The discriminating ability of gastric acid secretory tests in the diagnosis of recurrence after truncal vagotomy and drainage for duodenal ulcer. *Scand J Gastroenterol* 1973; **8**: 483 – 9

Kronborg O. The assessment of completeness of vagotomy. *Surg Clin North Am* 1976; **56**: 1421 – 34

Butterfield DJ, Whitfield PF, Hobsley M. Changes in gastric secretion with time after vagotomy and the relationship to recurrent duodenal ulcer. *Gut* 1982; **23**: 1055 – 9

Maybury NK, Faber RG, Hobsley M. Post-vagotomy insulin test. *Gut* 1977; **18**: 449 – 56

Meldrum SJ, Watson BW, Riddle HC, Bown RL, Sladen GE. pH profile of gut as measured by radiotelemetry capsule. *Br Med J* 1972; **2**: 104 – 6

Fordtran JS, Walsh JH. Gastric acid secretion rate and buffer content of the stomach after eating. *J Clin Invest* 1973; **52**: 645 – 59

Taylor IL. Gastrointestinal hormones in peptic ulcer disease. *Clin Gastroenterol* 1984; **13**: 363 – 4

Pendower JEH. A comparison of the Burge and Grassi intra-operative tests for completeness of nerve section in parietal cell vagotomy. *Br J Surg* 1981; **68**: 83 – 4

OTHER GASTRIC SECRETIONS

It is possible to measure sodium, potassium, chloride, bicarbonate, calcium, pepsin, intrinsic factor, intrinsic factor antibodies, protein, lipase and amylase, mucus and viscosity in gastric juice. In practice the only technique much used is that for pepsin.

Pepsin

Pepsin is the gastric protease; it is secreted in parallel with acid which activates 80% of the gastric protease activity.

Method

Radioiodinated serum albumin (RISA) is used. Radioactive albumin is digested by gastric proteases to release the isotope which is then counted. Gastric juice which has been obtained by gastric aspiration without any stimulus is filtered through gauze. To 1 ml bovine albumin carrier 1 ml RISA is added and the pH is adjusted to 2 by adding about 3 ml of Sorensen's buffer. Then 1 ml of the clear gastric juice is added to the isotope solution and the mixture is incubated at 37°C for 15 min at which stage 1 ml 50% trichloracetic acid is added. The precipitate is centrifuged and the clear supernate is counted for 1 min in a scintillation counter. The radioactivity is converted into mg pepsin/ml.

Interpretation

The normal range is 0.15 – 1.0 mg pepsin/ml.

Vitamin B_{12} urinary excretion (Schilling) test)

This test is frequently performed in two parts, thereby testing both the ability of the gastric mucosa to secrete intrinsic factor and the ability of the terminal ileum to absorb vitamin B_{12}. The isotope that is usually used is ^{58}Co-B_{12} which should be stored in the refrigerator.

Method

Part 1. After an overnight fast the patient empties the bladder and the urine is discarded. 0.5 – 1.0 mcCi radioactive vitamin B_{12} is taken orally in 50 ml water and a flushing dose of 1000 mcg of non-radioactive vitamin B_{12} administered intramuscularly in order to saturate the body stores. All urine voided is collected for 24 hours. The urine is sent to the isotope laboratory where a 5 ml aliquot is counted and compared with a standard of radioactive vitamin B_{12} prepared from the stock from which the test dose has been taken.

Part 2. The second part of the test should not be undertaken within 3 days of performing Part 1. After an overnight fast the bladder is emptied and the urine discarded. The radioactive vitamin B_{12} is administered orally as before together with a capsule of 50 mg intrinsic factor and this is followed by the intramuscular flushing dose of non-radioactive vitamin B_{12}. Urine is then collected and tested for radioactivity as in Part 1. A reticulocyte count is usually taken daily for 2 – 3 days following the injection.

Interpretation

The results are expressed as a percentage of the dose ingested. Normally 10% or more of the dose is excreted in the urine during the first 24 hours. A low value in Part 1 suggests either an absence of intrinsic factor or defective absorption of vitamin B_{12} by the terminal ileum. The administration of intrinsic factor improves the absorption of vitamin B_{12} in Addisonian pernicious anaemia. Low values are also found in the blind loop syndrome and jejunal diverticulosis but values are usually higher (2–7%) than in Addisonian pernicious anaemia (0–3%).

A low value of excretion in Part 2 of the test which is similar to Part 1 suggests that the terminal ileum is diseased or absent.

This is a simple and reliable test but there are disadvantages such as the problems of obtaining a complete 24-hour urine collection and the results are inaccurate in the presence of inadequate renal function. The reproducibility of the test is poor particularly after partial gastrectomy, with diffuse small bowel disease and with bacterial invasion of the gut. The test procedure may be varied in the dose of radioactivity given, the dose of the flushing injection of non-radioactive vitamin B_{12} and the duration of urine collection which should be for 48 hours if there is renal impairment.

A useful modification of this test is the Dicopac method in which intrinsic-factor bound B_{12} and free B_{12} are given simultaneously. Each of the two B_{12} fractions is labelled with different isotopes of cobalt (^{57}Co and ^{58}Co) and the urine is analysed by differential counting to give equivalent results to Parts 1 and 2 of the Schilling test.

Serum vitamin B_{12}

Normal results are from 200–800 pg/ml. Values are *very low* in pernicious anaemia, *low* in bacterial overgrowth of the gut and intestinal hurry, and often *high* in parenchymal or neoplastic liver disease.

Gastric antibodies

Antibodies directed against the parietal cells and intrinsic factor may be present in both gastric juice and serum.

Parietal cell antibodies

These can be demonstrated by conventional immunological techniques such as complement fixation and the immunofluorescent test using rabbit antihuman gamma-globulin fluorescein conjugate. About 10% of 'normal' subjects and 60–90% of patients with Addisonian pernicious anaemia have circulating parietal cell antibodies. Parietal cell antibodies are never found in the presence of a normal gastric mucosa; their presence in serum or gastric juice suggests chronic gastritis and is associated with some reduction in gastric acid output. They may be present in patients with chronic gastritis who do not have pernicious anaemia. On the other hand patients with advanced chronic gastritis may have no parietal cell antibodies.

Intrinsic factor antibodies

Antibodies to intrinsic factor are rarely found in normal sera. About 30–50% of patients with Addisonian pernicious anaemia have antibodies against intrinsic factor, but the patients differ in the type of antibody present. The antibodies correlate with an advanced degree of gastric atrophy and are associated with some degree of abnormality of vitamin B_{12} absorption. Large doses of vitamin B_{12} given intramuscularly within 48 hours of testing the serum can cause false-positive tests for intrinsic factor antibodies.

Gastric cytology

Exfoliative cytology is of great value in the diagnosis of gastric lesions, particularly cancer. In many centres this investigation is provided as a routine service.

The use of the cytology brush at endoscopy combined with examination of the smears by experienced cytologists is claimed to yield better results than the histology of endoscopic biopsies. Additional material may be obtained by washing the endoscope after the examination with 200 ml physiological saline, which yields tens of thousands of cells.

Cytological interpretation is said to be easy in about 80% of gastric cancers. Gastric Hodgkin's disease and lymphosarcoma can also be diagnosed from the smears. The method is reliable and false-positive results need not exceed 0.5%. It is probably the most accurate method of establishing a preoperative diagnosis of gastric cancer and is of particular value when deformities of the fundus or antrum are present. Failures in diagnosis are due uncommonly to faulty interpretation and are more probably the consequence of inadequate cell collection.

Fluorescence cytology

The cells of gastric cancers form complexes with tetracycline and these

47

demonstrate fluorescence under ultraviolet light. This property has been utilized in a diagnostic test for gastric malignant disease.

Method

Tetracycline 500 mg daily is taken orally for 2–4 days. Thirty-six hours after the last dose exfoliative cytology is performed on the fasting patient. After collection the aspirate is neutralized with 5% sodium bicarbonate solution to bring the pH to 7–9, centrifuged at 3000 rpm for 10 min and the sediment spread thinly over filter paper. The paper is examined immediately on drying and again 24 hours later in a dark room using ultraviolet light.

Interpretation

Normal cells show no fluorescence. Specks of blue represent mucosal cells and this is not abnormal. Malignant cells show bright yellow fluorescence and exfoliated lymphomatous cells also give a positive fluorescence. The test is reported to show a high degree of accuracy with about 7% of false-positive results. The presence of pyloric obstruction, even if it is partial, may give false-positive results, and it has been suggested that the tetracycline should be given intramuscularly in a dose of 250 mg twice a day for 2 days when there is gastric retention. Failure to neutralize the gastric aspirate will cause false-negative results because the tetracycline will not fluoresce in a strongly acid pH.

Reference

Sandlow LJ, Allen HA, Necheles H. The use of tetracycline fluorescence in the detection of gastric malignancy. *Ann Intern Med* 1963; **58**: 401–13

Gastric biopsy

This is conveniently performed with the endoscope biopsy forceps.

Interpretation

The *normal* stomach has variable architecture, and it is necessary to take biopsies from stated and standardized positions to enable proper interpretation. One biopsy from the antrum, two from different parts of the greater curve and one from the mid-lesser curve provide a fair sampling procedure.

It is not usually worth taking biopsies from the cardia unless there is macroscopic disease.

Acute gastritis is characterized by infiltration of leucocytes, mucosal haemorrhages and erosions. It may be patchy so that biopsy appearances do not always correlate with endoscopy appearances.

Chronic gastritis may result from pyloric reflux or from gastric surgery, or other causes which may not be identifiable. Its relationship with symptoms and with gastric ulcer remains doubtful. In the initial stage it is probably accompanied by gastric acid hypersecretion, but eventually hyposecretion supervenes. Whether this is cause or effect is contentious.

The histological classification is based on four features.

(1) *Mucosal type*:

  (a) Pyloric (antral)
  (b) Body
  (c) Cardiac
  (d) Transitional
  (e) Indeterminate.

  In severe gastritis atrophy or metaplasia may occur, and the whole gastric mucosa may resemble the antral glandular structure or even the small intestinal architecture.

(2) *Grade*:

  (a) *Superficial gastritis* affects only the superficial, epithelium, gastric pits and related lamina propria.
  (b) *Atrophic gastritis* results in destruction of the glands and this may be determined by reticulin stains. This is graded as mild, moderate or severe.

(3) *Activity*:

  (a) Quiescent
  (b) Active

  Infiltration with polymorphonuclear leucocytes and epithelial degeneration indicates activity.

(4) *Metaplasia*:

  (a) *Intestinal metaplasia* nearly always occurs in association with atrophic gastritis.

(b)   *Pseudo-pyloric* or *antral metaplasia* is often found in atrophic gastritis.

In *pernicious anaemia* a different pattern is seen: the stomach is involved in an autoimmune gastritis characterized by an intensely cellular atrophic mucosa containing many lymphocytes and plasma cells.

Carcinoma is usually recognized macroscopically, but carcinoma-in-situ is well recognized to occur in ostensibly normal mucosa. The epithelium also may appear normal in leather-bottle stomach, when adequate histology is diagnostic. *Cellular atypia* is sometimes reported but its significance is even less certain than such changes in the colon. The extent of gastric carcinoma may be assessed by spraying the stomach with congo red at endoscopy or operation (non-carcinomatous acid-secreting areas appear black) or by pre-treatment of patients with toluidine blue.

References

Whitehead R, Truelove S, Gear MWL. The histological diagnosis of chronic gastritis in fibreoptic gastroscope biopsy specimens. *J Clin Pathol* 1972; **25**: 1–11
Hallisey MT, Fielding JWL. *In vivo* stain for gastric cancer. *Lancet* 1988; **1**: 115

Radiology (Figure 10)

Gastric radiology is a most important method for examining the stomach.

Gastric ulcers and benign and malignant tumours

Differentiation between benign and malignant gastric ulcer may be difficult. Some of the important features of a malignant gastric ulcer are rigid angular margins to the ulcer, a long shallow irregular ulcer having irregular edges, an ulcer lying within the line of the gastric profile, a clear zone separating the ulcer from the barium in the stomach and the barium-filled crater, irregular translucency around the base and the disappearance of the ulcer with no lessening of the surrounding rigidity. Criteria which are of little help in the differentiation of benign from malignant ulcers are the site and size of the ulcer, the appearance of the rugal folds and any shortening of the lesser curvature. Carcinomas may also appear as polyps or diffuse infiltration (leather bottle stomach).

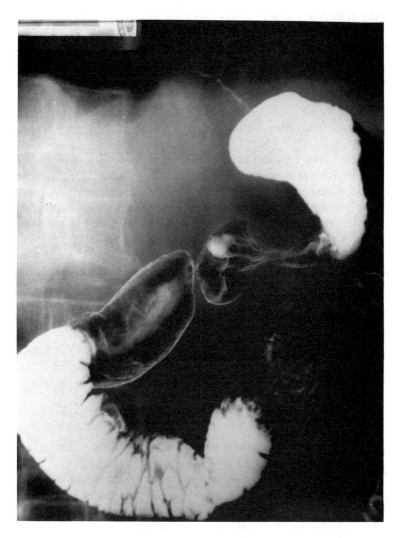

Figure 10 Barium meal showing leather bottle stomach (diffuse carcinoma)

Gastritis

The radiological diagnosis of the various forms is difficult and controversial. Acute gastritis, gastric erosions and probably chronic gastritis are not usually associated with characteristic radiological features. Atrophic gastritis and gastric atrophy are said to have recognisable features including a long tubular stomach, the absence of rugal markings on the greater curvature and a 'bald' fundus.

Duodenal ulcer

The barium meal is most important in diagnosis, but it may be very difficult to make the diagnosis of active ulceration in the presence of a scarred duodenal cap.

Iodinated water-soluble opaque media

These (e.g. 'Gastrografin') are justifiably unpopular with many radiologists. Such materials are hypertonic and are markedly diluted in the bowel to give very poor contrast. They are dangerous in the dehydrated patient, particularly infants. Barium is of more value when ileus or obstruction is present. In an emergency where much vomiting is present and inhalation is feared, it is still better to use a dilute barium suspension than other media.

However, the water-soluble opaque agents are recommended when perforation is suspected because extravasation of these media is harmless.

Double-contrast radiology

The introduction of the double-contrast barium meal, in which effervescent tablets or carbonated drinks are used, has improved diagnostic accuracy. Mucosal lesions can be identified much more readily, and in the hands of enthusiasts overall accuracy can equal that of endoscopy.

Computed tomography and magnetic resonance imaging

CT and MRI are useful secondary procedures for gauging the extent and operability of gastric, and more especially of gastro-oesophageal and oesophageal carcinomas.

Not only can the size and position of tumours be assessed, but also the presence of metastases in nodes, liver and lung.

Campylobacter-like organisms (CLO)

These are found in the gastric antrum in a high proportion of patients with gastritis and peptic ulcer disease, and are also found in a high proportion of those with healed peptic ulcer disease destined to relapse. However, the organisms are common with advancing age in healthy people, and the significance for management of individual patients is unclear.

(1) The spiral organisms with bulb-ended flagella can be identified on light or electron microscopy in biopsy samples of gastric antrum. Monoclonal antibodies can be used to provide rapid immunofluorescent detection: gram stains may be sufficient.

(2) Culture of gastric antral biopsies under micraerophilic conditions on chocolate agar or Oxoid BAB with Skirrow's formula will confirm the presence of CLO.

(3) The potent urease activity of CLO can be used in a number of ways. Simply putting an infected biopsy in freshly prepared 10% urea in deionised water at pH 6.8 with two drops of 1% phenol red will produce a colour change from orange-yellow to red-pink in 1 – 10 min. Urease activity can be demonstrated after microbiological culture or by an isotope-labelled urea breath test.

(4) Enzyme-linked immunosorbent assay (ELISA) based on CLO-specific urease antigen can be used as a serum test in infected patients.

References

Rokkas T, Sladen GE. Infection with *Campylobacter pylori*. *J R Coll Physicians London* 1988; **22**: 97–100

Arvinda S, Cook RS, Tabaqchali S, Farthing MJG. One-minute endoscopy room test for *Campylobacter pylori*. *Lancet* 1988; **1**: 704

Dent JC, McNulty CAM, Uff JS, Gear MWL, Wilkinson SP. *Campylobacter pylori* urease. A new serological test. *Lancet* 1988; **1**: 1002

CHAPTER 6

Absorption

Major causes of persistent steatorrhoea are coeliac disease, chronic pancreatic disease including cystic fibrosis, pancreatic carcinoma and gastric surgery. There are many other causes, and acute self-limiting steatorrhoea is a common feature of infective gastroenteritis and acute pancreatitis.

FATS AND RELATED SUBSTANCES

Triolein breath test (Figure 11)

Because of the practical problems of faecal fat estimation various isotope tests have been proposed. The most satisfactory test is the triolein breath test (Figure 11). This test is best avoided in patients with respiratory disease. Glyceryl-^{14}C-triolein is given with a carrier meal and breath $^{14}CO_2$ activity is counted. Each of the three oleic acid molecules is labelled with ^{14}C. The basis of the test is that the oleic acid is absorbed after digestion of triglyceride, and metabolized in the body to CO_2 and H_2O.

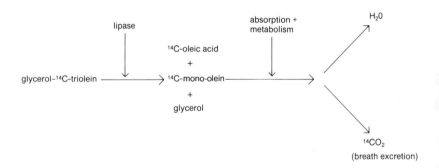

Figure 11 Triolein breath test

Method

The patient is studied while eating a normal diet and while avoiding drugs which affect intestinal mobility.

After an overnight fast 5 mcCi glyceryl-^{14}C-triolein is given by mouth with a standard 20 g liquid fat meal. Breath is collected before the test meal and hourly for 6 hours afterwards. Patients are asked to exhale through a rubber tube connected to a Pasteur pipette, the end of which is under the surface of the trapping solution. This contains 2 mmol of a quarternary amine (hyamine hydroxide) in ethanol with thymolphthalein as indicator. The patients continue bubbling their exhaled gas through until the indicator turns from blue to colourless, when 2 mmol CO_2 has been trapped. $^{14}CO_2$ is then measured in each of the samples by liquid scintillation counting, and the output of $^{14}CO_2$ is expressed as percentage dose excreted per hour.

Interpretation

The best separation of steatorrhoea from normal is found by taking the result for the period when $^{14}CO_2$ excretion is maximal. This peak $^{14}CO_2$ excretion is less than 3.5% in steatorrhoea and greater than 3.5% in normals.

The value at 6 hours after ingestion of the test meal gives similar but slightly inferior results. If all the results are cumulated, normal controls excrete more than 9% of the administered dose, whereas in steatorrhoea less than 6% is excreted. The test is dependent on body mass, and can give false-positive results in obesity.

Indications

This test is useful when it is necessary to monitor steatorrhoea in a patient. It has been recommended as a preliminary screening test to reduce the number of faecal fat estimations.

A modification using ^{13}C-triolein and measuring breath $^{13}CO_2$ by mass spectroscopy is being developed to avoid the use of radioisotope, but is unlikely to be widely useful because of the costly equipment required.

References

Newcomer AD, Hofmann AF, DiMagno EP, Thomas PJ, Carlson GL. Triolein breath test. *Gastroenterology* 1979; **76**: 6–13

Mylvaganam K, Hudson PR, Ross A, Williams CP. ^{14}C-triolein breath test: a routine test in the gastroenterology clinic? *Gut* 1986; **27**: 1347–52

Watkins JB, Klein PD, Schoeller DA, Kirschner BS, Park R, Derman JA. Diagnosis and differentiation of fat malabsorption in children using ^{13}C-labelled lipids; trioctanoin, triolein and palmitic acid breath tests. *Gastroenterology* 1982; **82**: 911–7

West PS, Levin GE, Griffin GE, Maxwell JD. Comparison of simple screening tests for fat malabsorption. *Br Med J* 1981; **282**: 1501–4

Faecal fat excretion

Fat is present in the faeces in three forms: as neutral fat (triglycerides, 'unsplit' fat); free fatty acids ('split' fat); and sodium, potassium and calcium salts of the fatty acids (soaps). The origin of the faecal fat is not fully understood. It is in part exogenous, being derived from unabsorbed dietary fat, but also partly endogenous from the bile, desquamated cells and the breakdown of bacteria.

Method

It is important that the patient is eating a normal diet; patients with steatorrhoea often control diarrhoea by reducing fat intake. Patients should be told that satisfactory results depend on diet, and it is worthwhile arranging a consultation with the dietician to ensure an adequate intake.

The faeces excreted over a period of 3 or 5 consecutive days are collected and sent to the laboratory. The samples should be in clearly labelled and dated containers. If the patient is constipated a longer period of collection may be undertaken and this must be made clear to the laboratory. Periods of collection shorter than 3 days are unsatisfactory and inaccurate, as the amount of fat contained in a single stool specimen can vary widely.

Plastic, radio-opaque, or dye markers can be used to ensure complete collection for a given number of days. The faeces should be uncontaminated by barium and the patient must not be taking castor oil. Liquid paraffin does not affect the neutral fat level when the van de Kamer method is used.

The collection of stools should present no problems *in hospital* where the stools passed into bedpans can be transferred to labelled tins. The *outpatient* collection of stools is much more difficult and uncertain. The following technique has been suggested for outpatients. A polythene sheet is cut into the shape of a wide-mouthed cone 24 inches in diameter. This can be held conveniently in place between the seat and the basin of the lavatory, and after defecation the sheet and faeces are transferred to a container. One can is used for each day and at the end of the day the lid is sealed with adhesive tape. It is desirable but not essential that the cans are stored in a refrigerator until analysis.

In the laboratory the stool is mixed with water, homogenized, and the collection pooled. After thorough mixing, a 10 ml aliquot is analysed by hydrolysis, extraction and titration of the fatty acids. The result may be expressed as fatty acids but is usually expressed as amount of neutral fat excreted per day.

Interpretation

The normal maximum daily output of fat is 18 mmol or about 7 g in adults, but the upper limits vary in different laboratories. A patient who excretes more than the normal daily amount of fat in the stool is said to have steatorrhoea. There is very little difference in the amount of fat excreted in the stool when normal subjects take diets varying between 50–250 g fat/day but in patients with malabsorption the stool fat content is more closely related to the dietary fat intake. The ordinary mixed diet in the United Kingdom contains 70–90 g fat/day.

No markers are required in this test. The method gives poor recovery of short- and medium-chain fatty-acid triglycerides. This is normally not a problem as the average diet contains almost exclusively the long-chain triglycerides, but some artificial diets contain fat as medium-chain triglycerides which do not require digestion prior to absorption. Markers such as cuprous thiocyanate, carmine or radio-opaque pellets have been used to ensure complete collections. In theory this is an attractive method, but it is handicapped by the fact that luminal contents are not homogenous and that solids, oils and aqueous solutes travel at different rates.

Indications

The faecal fat output is a widely used index of the state of digestion and absorption in the small intestine. Steatorrhoea is a feature of a number of diseases involving the small intestine, the pancreas, the hepatobiliary system, and also in many patients who have had a partial gastrectomy or a vagotomy and drainage procedure. The terms steatorrhoea and malabsorption are frequently used interchangeably. Steatorrhoea implies only an excess of fat in the stool, but the presence of steatorrhoea is usually one of the cardinal features of malabsorption in which fluid, electrolytes, vitamins, carbohydrates and proteins may be poorly absorbed.

Macroscopic

The macroscopic appearance of a stool containing excess fat is sometimes characteristic: bulky, yellow or grey, soft and sticky with a rancid odour. The stool may be liquid, frothy and have floating oil droplets. On the other hand the stool may appear perfectly normal or even rather small and hard. Stools float in water because of increased gas content, which does not correlate with fat content.

Stool weight

The stool weight in Britain ranges normally up to a limit of 250 g/day. Steatorrhoea is unlikely but not impossible if the stool weight is less than 80 g/day. A clinically useful guide to the severity of steatorrhoea is obtained by weighing the stool daily, even though the correlation between the stool fat content and the stool weight is not close. By following progress in this way it is possible to avoid overburdening the laboratory with frequent requests for faecal fat estimation.

References

Van der Kamer JH, Huinink H, Ten B, Weyers HA. Rapid method for the determination of fat in faeces. *J Biol Chem* 1949; **177**: 347–55

Drummey GD, Benson JR Jr, Jones CM. Microscopical examination of the stool for steatorrhoea. *N Engl J Med* 1961; **264**: 85–87

Pryke ES, Whyte HM. A genteel device for collecting faeces. *Gut* 1970; **11**: 966

Moore JG, Englert E, Bigler AH, Clark RW. Simple fecal tests for absorption. A prospective survey and critique. *Am J Dig Dis* 1971; **16**: 97–105

Lee MF, Temperley JM, Dick M. Estimation of faecal fat excretion using cuprous thiocyanate as a continuous marker. *Gut* 1969; **10**: 754–9

Pedersen NT, Halgreen H. Faecal fat and faecal weight. *Scand J Gastroenterol* 1984; **19**: 350–54

Prothrombin time (PR, BCR, INR)

This reflects vitamin K absorption as well as liver synthesis. If the prothrombin time is more than 3 seconds longer than control, and reverts to normal after treatment for 3 days with vitamin K 10 mg i.m. or i.v. daily, then vitamin K malabsorption is established. This may accompany any cause of steatorrhoea. An INR of 1.3 or less gives equivalent information.

Serum vitamin D (25-hydroxy vitamin D)

In addition to dietary sources of vitamin D, there is an appreciable synthesis in the skin under the influence of daylight. Low values may be found in inadequate vitamin D intake and in individuals (especially with pigmented skins) who are not exposed to sufficient daylight. Values are markedly seasonal with higher values in summer.

The normal adult range of values is 25–75 nmol/l in summer and 15–60 nmol/l in winter. Some laboratories can separate 25-OH-ergocalciferol (dietary origin), low in malabsorption, from 25-OH-cholecalciferol (endogenous synthesis).

Vitamin A absorption

The fasting patient is given 7500 iu vitamin A/kg (maximum 350,000 iu) in 7 ml peanut oil and with a standard light breakfast.

Blood is taken before and at 4, 5 and 6 hours after the vitamin dose. Normal diet is allowed after the 4-hour sample. All blood samples are protected from the light by taking them into tubes covered with silver paper, and storing in the dark until analysis. The serum vitamin A level may be conveniently measured by fluorimetry.

The normal fasting serum vitamin A is 0.8 – 5.4 mcmol/l, and the maximum increase after vitamin A is 6 – 61.7 mcmol/l. In malabsorption many of the fasting values fall in the normal range but the maximum increase is less than 6 mcmol/l. This test is unreliable in pancreatic disease, though average values are reduced.

Oxalate loading test

Patients with steatorrhoea have excessive absorption of dietary oxalate. Measurement of urinary oxalate after an oral oxalate load can be used as a screening test for steatorrhoea. Patients are given a standard diet containing 50 g fat, 1 g calcium and 30 mg oxalate for a week. On the last 3 days of this diet they are given sodium oxalate 300 mg twice daily with meals, and on the last day a 24-hour urine collection is made. Patients with steatorrhoea excrete more than 0.44 mmol oxalate/24 hours. Hyperoxaluria may also occur in patients with bile acid malabsorption. The test cannot be used in patients with substantially diseased or resected large intestine, as the colon is the main site of oxalate absorption.

Reference

Rampton DS, Kasidas GP, Rose GA, Sarner M. Oxalate loading test: a screening test for steatorrhoea. *Gut* 1979; **20**: 1089 – 94

Bile acid malabsorption

Some uncommon forms of diarrhoea are caused by excessive loss of bile acids into the colon from the small intestine. This can be measured by giving [75]selenium-labelled tauro-homocholic acid ([75]SeHCAT) by mouth, and measuring retention in the body. Normal conservation of bile acids in the enterohepatic circulation means that at 24 hours 80% of activity is retained in the body, 50% at 72 hours, and 15% or more at 7 days. A convenient test is to scan the patient's whole body with a gamma camera at 1 week to separate pathologically low retention from normal.

Though theoretically attractive this test confers no definite advantage over a therapeutic trial of bile-acid binding resin such as cholestyramine or colestipol.

References

Mahlstedt J. [75]SeHCAT-test – Indication and value in clinical diagnosis. *Der Nuklearmediziner* 1987; **10**: 183–96
Merrick MV, Eastwood MA, Ford MJ. Is bile acid malabsorption underdiagnosed? An evaluation of accuracy of diagnosis by measurement of SeHCAT retention. *Br Med J* 1985; **290**: 665–8

Other tests

The fat tolerance test can measure triglyceridaemia and chylomicronaemia after a standard meal. It depends on gastric emptying and clearance and metabolism of chylomicrons as well as fat malabsorption. It is not useful in individual patients.

Serum cholesterol and triglycerides tend to be lower in steatorrhoea, but values are too variable in controls to make this very useful.

In the rare condition abetalipoproteinaemia the serum cholesterol is extremely low and may be unrecordable with standard techniques. Lipoprotein electrophoresis shows an absent beta-lipoprotein band.

MONOSACCHARIDES

Xylose excretion

Xylose is a pentose sugar which is absorbed in the jejunum and excreted unchanged in the urine. The original xylose absorption test depended markedly on renal function and age. Results may be spuriously low in ascites. There has been a range of administered doses (5, 15 and 25 g), and xylose has been measured in both urine and blood. Results are often so difficult to interpret that many gastroenterologists have abandoned the test altogether.

If it is to be used in diagnosis then the method described by Haeney is the most attractive, though a ^{14}C-xylose breath test has been described as an investigation especially useful in small intestinal bacterial overgrowth.

Method

The patient is fasted overnight, apart from fluids which are encouraged. Height and weight are measured and surface area is derived from *Geigy Scientific Tables*. After a baseline blood sample has been taken to estimate non-xylose reducing component, D-xylose 5 g in 250 ml water is drunk quickly. Venous blood is sampled 1 hour later.

Interpretation

The result is corrected for surface area by the formula:

corrected blood value =

$$\text{measured value} \times \frac{\text{actual surface area}}{\text{constant ideal surface area (1.73)}}$$

The normal corrected value is 0.65–1.33 mmol/l, and patients with malabsorption have values below this.

Indications

(1) A screening test for steatorrhoea caused by small bowel disease.
(2) To measure jejunal absorptive capacity in monitoring disease progress.
(3) As a test for carbohydrate absorption.
(4) To distinguish between maldigestion (where food is not broken down normally and hence cannot be absorbed though absorptive capacity is normal) and malabsorption without maldigestion.

Oral glucose tolerance test

This has limited application, and should not be used in patients known to be diabetic. Blood glucose levels must be taken at defined intervals in relation to meals, and the patient must have been eating a normal diet during the 3 days before the test.

Method

Fasting blood is taken into an oxalate bottle for blood glucose estimation and a further sample is taken 2 hours after a normal breakfast.

If the fasting plasma glucose is greater than 8 mmol/l or the postprandial plasma glucose is greater than 11 mmol/l the patient has diabetes mellitus and no further test is useful. If not then a formal glucose tolerance test may be useful, and should be performed on a separate day:

(1)   a fasting blood sample is taken;
(2)   the patient quickly drinks 75 g glucose dissolved in 250 ml water;
(3)   blood glucose is sampled every 30 min for 2 hours;
(4)   urine is tested for sugar as often as conveniently possible.

Interpretation

A fasting plasma glucose >8 mmol/l or a plasma glucose >11 mmol/l 12 hours after glucose ingestion indicates diabetes mellitus. Glycosuria supports this but is often absent in the elderly. Diabetes mellitus develops in 15% of patients with acute pancreatitis, in 70% with chronic pancreatitis (almost always when there is steatorrhoea), and in 30% with pancreatic cancer.

When there is small bowel disease causing malabsorption there is a flattened curve in non-diabetic patients, and the blood glucose does not rise more than 2 mmol/l over fasting values. However, this can also be seen in normal subjects and where gastric emptying is slow.

Where gastric emptying is rapid, as after gastric surgery, the first blood glucose level will be high, 'alimentary hyperglycaemia', followed by very low levels which may produce symptoms. This occurs because of an inappropriately timed release of insulin. If this is suspected it is best to measure blood glucose every 10–15 min after the glucose load.

Disaccharides

The main disaccharidases in man are lactase, sucrase and maltase. Deficiency syndromes involving one or more of these disaccharidases have been described. Two forms of deficiency syndromes are recognized; a primary variety in which an isolated enzyme deficiency exists in an otherwise normal mucosa, and a secondary variety in which the disaccharide deficiency is only one of many enzymes which is lacking in a mucous membrane damaged from recognizable causes. By far the most common syndrome is one involving isolated lactase deficiency; this is frequent in Mediterranean and tropical countries but less common in northern Europe. It is more often seen in Negroes than Caucasians. Maltase and sucrase deficiencies are usually found in association with lactase deficiency, but infrequently occur in isolation and are then generally in children.

Lactose tolerance test

After an overnight fast the patient ingests 50 g lactose in 500 ml water. Venous blood samples are tested for glucose in the fasting state and every 30 min for 2 hours. A normal result is a rise in blood glucose of at least 1 mmol/l. A rise of less than this is considered to represent a flat absorption curve and is suggestive of lactase deficiency. Patients with normal lactase absorption curves usually have normal mucosal lactase activities. Lactose may be given in a dose of 1.5 g/kg body weight or, in children, as a dose of 50 g/m^2 of body surface. This test may also be performed using maltose or sucrose instead of lactose.

A tolerance test using 25 g glucose and 25 g galactose (the hydrolytic products of lactose) may be undertaken to confirm a diagnosis of lactase deficiency. Patients with lactase deficiency have a normal rise of blood glucose levels, and are symptom-free after ingesting the mixture of glucose and galactose, in contrast to the effects of a lactose load.

Symptomatology

Patients who have significant lactase deficiency will often develop abdominal cramps, distension, flatulence and diarrhoea 1–6 hours after ingesting 50 g lactose. At such time the stools may contain both lactic and acetic acids which result in a low stool pH of below 4 (normal pH is 7). However, an acid stool is not invariably present, particularly in adults. While the development of symptoms after 50 g lactose suggests lactase deficiency, the failure to react does not exclude intestinal lactase deficiency but implies only that the clinical syndrome is absent. Fifty grams is the approximate lactose content of a litre of milk and this volume can be used as test dose, instead of the refined sugar.

Intestinal disaccharidase activity

After an overnight fast a jejunal biopsy is performed at or beyond the ligament of Treitz using either a Crosby capsule or the multipurpose suction biopsy tube. The biopsy specimen is orientated on filter paper and divided into two portions, one for histology and the other for enzyme estimation. The latter portion is immediately frozen on dry ice or liquid nitrogen.

It is best to measure the activity of all three disaccharides which is done by incubation with the appropriate disaccharide substrate at 37°C for 1 hour and measuring the glucose liberated. The results are expressed in mcmol/g wet weight of tissue/min (or at mcmol/g protein/min).

Normal ranges are for lactase 2.0–7.0 mcmol/g/min, for sucrase 2.5–9 mcmol/g/min, and for maltase 8.5–3 mcmol/g/min. There is no alteration with age. Activities are lower in the stomach and duodenum, so accurate positioning of the capsule is essential.

Lactase activity below normal in the presence of normal maltase and sucrase activity indicates lactase deficiency. This may be primary or secondary to other bowel disorders. If all three enzyme activities are low the patient is unlikely to have primary lactase deficiency and the cause is probably secondary to other bowel disorders. In symptomatic lactase malabsorption, lactase activity is probably uniformly absent throughout the whole of the small intestine.

The syndrome of lactase intolerance was first recognized in children, but it is now apparent that symptoms may manifest for the first time in adult life. The prevalence of isolated lactase deficiency in symptom-free individuals is still uncertain. The results of population surveys have varied, some suggesting that selective lactase deficiency occurs in 30 – 55% of individuals while other studies suggest that only 15% of subjects have the enzyme deficiency.

Secondary depression of intestinal lactase activity is found in diseases of the small intestinal mucosa such as coeliac disease, tropical sprue, giardiasis and a number of other malabsorption states. Reduced enzyme activity has also been recorded in inflammatory bowel disease. Lactase is the first of the three important intestinal disaccharidases to be reduced in the presence of small intestine disease.

Indications

A test for lactase activity is indicated in patients with a history of milk intolerance, unexplained abdominal cramps and diarrhoea. When patients with coeliac disease or the irritable bowel colon syndrome fail to respond to conventional therapy or respond only poorly, removing lactose-containing foods from the diet may produce considerable symptomatic relief, hence documentation of the enzyme deficiency is advantageous.

Other tests

Disaccharidase deficiency states may be demonstrated by mixing 25 g of the appropriate sugar (lactose, sucrose or maltose) with the barium suspension and screening the patient. Patients who have an enzyme deficiency show dilution of the contrast medium, rapid transit time and dilatation of the bowel lumen.

Hydrogen breath test

It has been shown that patients with disaccharidase deficiency excrete more hydrogen and less CO_2 after an appropriate disaccharide load. Thus in the first 3 hours after 12 g lactose by mouth, patients with lactase deficiency excrete more than 20 ppm. of hydrogen in the breath, whereas healthy individuals excrete less than 4 ppm. This test is simple but not widely used. Methane is not always present in breath and its measurement is an unhelpful test.

References

King CE, Toskes PP. Comparison of the 1g ^{14}C-xylose, 10 g lactulose-H_2, and 80 g glucose-H_2 breath tests in patients with small intestine bacterial overgrowth. *Gastroenterology* 1986; **91**: 1447–51

Haeney MR, Culank LS, Montgomery RD, Sammons HG. Evaluation of xylose as measured in blood and urine. A one-hour blood xylose screening test in malabsorption. *Gastroenterology* 1978; **75**: 393–400

Diem K, Lentner G. *Geigy Scientific Tables*. Basle: Geigy

Trinder P. Micro-determination of xylose in plasma. *Analyst* 1975; **100**: 12–15

Howell JN, Mellmann J, Ehlers P, Flatz G. Intestinal disaccharidase activities and activity ratios in a group of 60 German subjects. *Hepatogastroenterology* 1980; **27**: 208–12

National Diabetes Data Group. Classification and diagnosis of diabetes mellitus and other categories of glucose tolerance. *Diabetes* 1979; **28**: 1039–57

Ladas S, Papanikos J, Arapakis G. Lactose malabsorption in Greek adults. *Gut* 1982; **23**: 968–73

Ferguson A. Diagnosis and treatment of lactose intolerance. *Br Med J* 1981; **283**: 1423–24

Editorial. When does lactose malabsorption matter in adults? *Br Med J* 1975; **ii**: 351–52

HAEMATINICS

Vitamin B_{12}

Serum B_{12} levels are low in many diseases causing malabsorption, often because of intestinal hurry. This is non-specific. However, low serum B_{12} is commonly due to other causes such as pernicious anaemia. A two-part Schilling test (or use of the Dicopac modification) can demonstrate the inability of the terminal ileum to absorb B_{12}–intrinsic factor complexes; it is therefore a useful test of terminal ileal function.

Folic acid absorption

Folic acid is absorbed in the jejunum. In addition to dietary sources (mainly as polyglutamates) folic acid may be synthesized by intestinal bacteria, and in this way elevated serum levels can occur.

The patient is saturated with folic acid by a daily intramuscular injection of 15 mg folic acid for 3 days. Thirty-six hours after the last injection, and after an overnight fast, a blood sample is obtained and this is followed by an oral dose of 40 mcg folic acid/kg body weight. Blood samples are obtained 1 and 2 hours later, and serum folic acid levels are measured. In normal subjects the peak serum concentration of folic acid is greater than 40 mcg/l. Values below this are abnormal and are found in coeliac disease and other diseases involving the upper small intestine. This is a pharmacological test and gives no information about the absorption of folic acid from dietary sources.

Iron absorption

Iron is normally absorbed from the duodenum, or from the first normal part of the small bowel which food enters after leaving the stomach. Iron deficiency is a common feature of many disorders of absorption of the small intestine, but also occurs frequently from deficient intake and blood loss. The blood film shows hypochromia and microcytosis, i.e. pale small red cells. The serum iron is low and iron-binding capacity is raised so that percentage saturation is below 15%. Serum ferritin levels correlate fairly well with body iron stores, and in iron deficiency are below 17 mcg/l.

Current methods utilize isotopically labelled iron preparations. Iron in the diet may be presented to the intestine in the inorganic form (when the salts are first reduced to the ferrous state) or else as haemoglobin iron which is absorbed as haem or possibly as the whole molecule. Thus the carrier iron for labelled preparations may be either labelled inorganic iron or labelled haemoglobin iron. The nature of the carrier iron may well influence the result, and it is probable that the amount of unlabelled carrier iron is also important.

Whole body counting

After an overnight fast 5–10 mcg Ci ^{59}Fe-labelled iron is given orally, (usually as ^{59}Fe-ferric chloride) in a meal containing 5–7 mg elemental iron. The isotope may be mixed with the meal or taken in 100 ml water during the meal. A whole body count is made 4 hours later. This value is taken to represent the 100% retention value. The final absorption count is made about 10–14 days later when any unabsorbed iron has been excreted. The results are expressed as a percent age of the initial dose absorbed. This test is probably the best test available; it is quick and simple for the patient and avoids stool collections.

Faecal recovery method

Inorganic iron. After an overnight fast the patient is given 5–10 mcCi ^{59}Fe usually as ferric chloride as described above.

Organic iron. ^{59}Fe-labelled rabbit haemoglobin is prepared. Ten millilitres of rabbit blood containing about 5 mcCi radioactive iron is made palatable by the addition of a flavouring agent and taken with a standard meal containing about 5 mg iron.

Stools are collected daily until less than 1% of the administered dose appears. Counting may take place in a ring of Geiger-Müller tubes or in a well-type scintillation counter if the stools are dried.

The results may be expressed in two ways, either as that percentage of the administered dose which is absorbed when the normal level is 8% with a range of 0–15%, or as the percentage of the administered dose appearing in the faeces when the normal is 87–100%.

Double isotope method

In this method ^{59}Fe iron is incubated with the patient's plasma and injected intravenously, while ^{55}Fe iron is given orally in a meal similar to that mentioned above. A blood sample is tested after 14 days, and the activities of the two isotopes are measured in the red cells by differential counting. The ^{59}Fe counts indicate the percentage of the plasma iron which is used for haemoglobin synthesis and the absorbed ^{55}Fe utilized for haemoglobin synthesis is assumed to be the same. The ratio of the two isotopes in a blood sample gives a measure of absorption which is normally between 1–13%. The accuracy of this test has been questioned, particularly in liver disease.

Interpretation

Malabsorption of some form of iron occurs in a significant proportion of patients with partial gastrectomy and also in coeliac disease. Absorption is normal in achlorhydria and increased in states with erythroid hyperplasia. At some stage in haemochromatosis, in porphyria cutanea tarda, and in some patients with chronic pancreatic disease, there is increased iron absorption.

References

Watson WS, Hume R, Moore MR. Oral absorption of lead and iron. *Lancet* 1980; **2**: 236–7

Chanarin I, Anderson BB, Mollin DL. The absorption of folic acid. *Br J Haematol* 1958; **4**: 156–66

Lunn JA, Richmond J, Simson JD, Leask JD, Tothill P. Comparison between 3 radioisotope methods for measuring iron absorption. *Br Med J* 1967; **3**: 331–3

OTHER TESTS FOR MALABSORPTION

There is no satisfactory method for measuring protein absorption because amino acids are partly catabolized and partly reused in protein synthesis, and also many gastrointestinal diseases are associated with protein exudation.

Radioisotope tests of absorption of various metal ions such as calcium and copper have been described but in practice have little diagnostic usefulness.

Rare disorders of intestinal absorption

There are a number of uncommon hereditary disorders involving the absorption of a variety of metabolites, and in many of these diarrhoea may be a prominent symptom.

Dibasic amino acids

There is a defect in the transport of lysine, ornithine, cystine and arginine in cystinuria. The intestinal defect may be demonstrated by a tolerance test to orally ingested arginine and also by peroral biopsies of the intestinal mucosa which show poor concentration of the dibasic amino acids.

Tryptophan

There is defective intestinal transport of this amino acid (mono-amino-mono-carboxylic) in Hartnup disease. The defect can be demonstrated by a tolerance test to orally administered tryptophan but the tryptophan load has not been standardized. There is also a reduced intestinal transport of tryptophan in phenylketonuria, maple syrup disease and isolated intestinal tryptophan malabsorption.

Methionine

In patients with isolated methionine malabsorption, 'oast-house syndrome', there is profuse diarrhoea after the ingestion of methionine and an excess of alpha-hydroxybutyric acid in the urine.

CHAPTER 7

Small intestine

The function of the small bowel can be evaluated by clinical tests of absorption (Chapter 6). Intestinal biopsy, bacteriology, radiology, radio-isotope studies and serology provide additional information to enable specific diagnoses to be made.

INTESTINAL BIOPSY

Endoscopic forceps biopsy

This is the standard procedure, since it is rapid and reliable. The best results are obtained by taking multiple biopsies of the distal duodenum with the largest available size of forceps. The duodenal bulb must not be used for non-targetted biopsy of apparently normal mucosa, but histological confirmation of visible abnormalities may occasionally be required.

The widest available channel endoscope should be used with the largest compatible forceps.

References

Scott BB, Jenkins D. Endoscopic small intestinal biopsy. *Gastrointest Endosc* 1981; **27**: 162 – 7
Mee AS, Burke M, Vallon AG, Newman J, Cotton PB. Small bowel biopsy for malabsorption: comparison of the diagnostic adequacy of endoscopic forceps and capsule biopsy specimens. *Br Med J* 1985; **291**: 769 – 72

Crosby – Kugler capsule

The instrument consists of a small capsule (9.5 x 18.5 mm) containing a rotating, spring-activated knife. In the wall of the capsule is a small port through which mucosa is drawn by suction. Suction also serves to trigger the knife which severs the mucosa and closes the port, thereby trapping a portion of the mucosa in the capsule. The capsule is attached to a 2 mm polyethylene catheter which serves both for holding the capsule and for suction.

Various modifications of the capsule have been proposed. If the tubing is replaced by a radio-opaque red arterial catheter the whole tube may be seen on the fluoroscope and loops identified and straightened: in addition this catheter is stiffer and allows progress by pushing the capsule onwards. Modern capsules have the spring secured in place by a steel plate which avoids the problem of loading. In practice the spring outlasts the life of the guillotine cylinder, and the usual limit on longevity is blunting of the cutting edge. Some capsules do not feature a retaining clip, some are supplied with a rubber jacket, and others are secured by a nut at the distal end which is tightened by an Allen key.

There are three methods for positioning the capsule.

Endoscopic

This is a rapid technique and takes minutes. The tubing should be about 50 cm longer than the endoscope, and it is necessary to check catheter length and diameter before commencing the intubation. The patient is prepared for a normal upper digestive endoscopy. The valve of a forward-viewing instrument is removed, the capsule is loaded and the Luer fitting removed from the proximal end of its tube. The capsule tubing is threaded retrogradely through the biopsy channel so that the capsule lies snugly against the distal tip of the endoscope. The endoscope is then passed in the usual way, with slight tension on the biopsy capsule catheter to keep the end closely applied to the endoscopic tip. The view is partially obscured, but it can be improved if necessary by advancing the capsule 2 cm from the end of the endoscope. The pylorus is located and the tip of the endoscope is held in position while 30 cm or more of the biopsy catheter is carefully advanced through the biopsy channel. The position of the biopsy capsule may be checked fluoroscopically but this is not necessary with experience. The Luer fitting is reattached. Five to ten millilitres of water followed by 10 ml air are flushed through the capsule tubing and the capsule is fired by applying suction; a 30 ml syringe is convenient for both of these purposes. The biopsy capsule is withdrawn to the tip of the endoscope and both removed together. The biopsy capsule is disassembled, the tissue sample floated in saline, examined by x10 hand lens or under a dissecting microscope, and quickly immersed in formol-saline. If enzyme studies are required the sample must be divided immediately and a portion frozen at once. Formalin inactivates disaccharides.

This method is fast, reliable and does not require fluoroscopy. It is, however, dependent on competent endoscopy. If upper gastrointestinal endoscopy is required in the same patient the instrument must be passed a second time and this is usually achieved without further medication.

Fluoroscopic method

The patient fasts overnight. The capsule is swallowed with the patient sitting forward and about 50 cm of tube passed. The patient then lies on the fluoroscopy bed, and it is confirmed that the tubing is not curling in the fundus of the stomach. If it is the capsule must be withdrawn to the cardia and a further attempt made at passage.

The patient is then asked to lie on the right side and the position of the capsule is checked periodically. Once it is estimated to have passed the pylorus it is pushed to the duodenojejunal flexure and fired. The technique often takes 1 hour or more, and various procedures have been proposed to facilitate it. A 100 cm outer polythene tube can be used to make the catheter more rigid until the capsule reaches the pylorus, and internal stiffening wires have been used for the same purpose. Another method is to give an intramuscular injection of 10–20 mg metoclopramide 10 min after swallowing the capsule. This agent relaxes sphincters and hurries the passage of the capsule into the stomach and duodenum.

The fluoroscopy method requires either a prolonged intubation or heavy commitment of the investigator's time with repeated fluoroscopy.

Traditional method

The capsule is swallowed 2 hours after the last meal of the day, which should be of light fluids. Thereafter only water is permitted. About 100 cm of tube is passed. The end of the tubing is attached to the cheek of the patient who is instructed to lie on the right side for a few hours. The following morning the patient is taken to the radiology department and the position of the capsule identified. Sometimes it will be found to have passed well beyond the ligament of Treitz. The capsule is withdrawn into the required position if necessary, biopsies usually being taken just beyond the duodenojejunal junction. If ileal biopsies are required more time and tube must be allowed for the capsule to pass down the intestine, and because the capsule is frequently not in the right position the examination may take days to complete.

Complications

The Crosby–Kugler is a safe instrument and complications from its use are very rare. The major hazard is intestinal perforation, which is particularly liable to occur in children. There is occasionally haemorrhage from the biopsy site and failure of the knife to sever a piece of mucosa completely may make it impossible to withdraw the capsule until the mucosal fragment has sloughed off. In the latter event patience is required from clinician and patient; the capsule generally frees itself within a day or two and can be recovered, usually with a sample too damaged for histological interpretation.

Rubin suction biopsy tube

In this instrument a cylindrical knife fits into a capsule which is in turn attached to a flexible tube. The capsule has a distal groove to which may be attached a finger-cot containing mercury. Different capsules are available containing one or more ports of different sizes, and special double knives are provided for use with the multi-hole capsules. The knife is attached to a pull wire which runs through the flexible tube and stationary handle, and it is attached to an activator handle. Suction is applied via a lateral arm on the stationary handle thereby drawing mucosa into the port. A vacuum gauge is attached to the handle so that the force of suction is measured, and this varies according to the age of the patient, the number of ports and the site of the biopsy. The capsule aperture is opened by pushing the activator handle (and therefore the knife) distally. The tube is passed with the knife positioned so that the port is closed. The procedure is best performed by two operators.

Method

After an overnight fast the patient is taken to the radiology department, the pharynx anaesthetized and the suction tube swallowed. The tube is positioned in the region of the pylorus under fluoroscopic control when there may be marked heaving and gastric contractions. The tube is then guided into the duodenum by gentle pressure. Alternatively the patient lies on the right lateral position for about 10 min, is re-screened and the procedure repeated until the tube is seen to have passed into the duodenum. Whether or not a small mercury bag attached to the capsule speeds progress is a matter of opinion. Many investigators feel that such an attachment hinders the passage of the tube.

Once in the duodenum the tube is usually readily positioned at the duodenojejunal flexure. The port is opened by pushing the knife forwards, suction is applied and a biopsy taken by traction on the activator handle. It is probably advisable to move the tube slightly and repeat the procedure to ensure that a biopsy is taken. The instrument is withdrawn with the knife in the closed position.

The instrument is safe and significant haemorrhage or perforation is rare.

The appreciation that upper small intestinal disease may be patchy has led to the popularity of the hydraulic instrument devised by Flick, which delivers biopsies immediately after they have been cut and allows multiple biopsies to be taken from multiple sites at one intubation.

A steerable catheter with a contoured distal Rubin biopsy capsule has been devised. It requires fluoroscopy for passage, and its advantage is the rapidity with which it can be manoeuvred into position.

The choice of the biopsy capsule and the technique depends on personal preference. With the Crosby capsule only one biopsy can be obtained, whereas the hydraulic capsule offers the possibility of an indefinite number. Smaller Crosby capsules are supplied for children.

Interpretation

Dissecting microscope

Normal appearance. The jejunal villi are long and finger-like and the vascular arcades are easily recognized. The height of a villus is about three times its width. Essentially similar features are found in the ileum. A normal variant is the broad, flat or leaf-shaped villus and this is seen particularly in duodenal biopsies where the leaves may even coalesce into ridges. An identical appearance may be seen in jejunal biopsy samples from normal subjects of Middle or Far Eastern extracion. These features may be identified with a hand lens.

Abnormalities. In coeliac disease the mucosal biopsy will be 'flat' or 'convoluted'. A 'flat' mucosa shows a complete loss of villi and the normal vascular arcades. There may be a mosaic or crazy pavement appearance. The 'convoluted' mucosa has no true villi but only ridges and whorls. While examination under the dissecting microscope or hand lens is a rapid and convenient diagnostic procedure it does not replace conventional histology. It is usually easy to recognize an abnormal villous pattern; the difficulty lies in deciding when villi are minimally abnormal. In this situation light microscopy is essential.

Light microscope

Normal appearance. Tall thin villi are seen lined by columnar epithelium. There are numerous goblet cells. Paneth and argentaffin cells may be seen at the base of the crypts of Lieberkühn. Mononuclear cells, plasma cells and eosinophils are seen in the lamina propria which is about one-half to one-third as thick as the villous height. Similar features are found in both finger- and leaf-shaped villi.

Brunner's glands are seen in the duodenum occupying the full thickness of the glandular (non-villus) mucosa. Villi may be blunted or absent. In the ileum more goblet cells are found, and the villi are slightly broader and shorter. There are collections of lymphoid cells, and villi overlying such areas are either stubby or absent. Specimens from apparently normal subjects in the Middle and Far East show a greater percentage of blunt and branched villi, more abnormal surface cells and slightly more prominent mononuclear cellular infiltration.

It is important to appreciate the variations in the appearance of the normal small bowel biopsy. The suggestion has been made that the 'finding of four adjacent villi *in any section* justifies an interpretation of normal villous architecture'.

Abnormalities. A number of diseases may be associated with minor non-specific abnormalities of the intestinal mucosa.

Coeliac disease. This is defined as the presence of total or subtotal villous atrophy which reverts to normal, or at least shows improvement, after the patient adheres to a gluten-free diet. It is important that milder abnormalities (partial villous atrophy) are not diagnosed as coeliac disease, because they are a common and non-specific finding.

Children with coeliac disease characteristically have total villous atrophy. There is virtual absence of the villi, thickening of the lamina propria, increased infiltration by lymphocytes and plasma cell, elongated crypts of Lieberkühn, increase in the mucosal glands and obvious surface epithelial abnormalities with increased intraepithelial lymphocytes. In less severe villous atrophy the villi are short, thickened and disorganized, the goblet cells are increased in number and there are lesser changes in the lamina propria. The mucosal changes in coeliac disease are seen maximally in the upper jejunum, but in severe involvement the changes will extend to the ileum. There is no correlation between the histological abnormalities and the absorptive function. A flat biopsy is found in some patients who do not respond to gluten withdrawal, and it is not possible to predict the response from the appearance of the intestinal biopsy. The typical appearance of coeliac disease may be found in the biopsies of patients who have, or will subsequently develop, intra-abdominal lymphomas or cancers of the gastro-intestinal tract.

Similar appearances can occur in dermatitis herpetiformis, and these sometimes respond to gluten exclusion. Psoriasis may occasionally be associated with villous atrophy.

Tropical sprue. The distinction between coeliac disease and tropical sprue is difficult morphologically because both demonstrate moderate to severe villous abnormalities. In tropical sprue the extent of the villous loss is marked and there are uniform small lipid droplets in the basement membrane adjacent to the surface epithelium.

Abetalipoproteinaemia (Acanthocytosis). There is normal villous architecture, but the intestinal cells are filled with fat-containing vacuoles.

Whipple's disease. The lamina propria is virtually replaced by macrophages filled with periodic acid-Schiff-positive glycoprotein granules. The normal villous architecture is distorted, and the lymphatics are dilated and filled with fat. Tiny bacilli can be seen with high-resolution light microscopy or with electron microscopy.

Agammaglobulinaemia. There is a complete absence of plasma cells. The villi may be near normal or totally atrophic, but the condition is readily differentiated from coeliac disease by this absence of plasma cells.

Other diseases. In the five conditions described above jejunal biopsy is invariably helpful. In some others, such as lymphangectasia, lymphoma, giardiasis, amyloidosis and Crohn's disease, biopsy may be helpful but is not necessarily so.

Non-specific changes include mild flattening and broadening of the villi, an increase in chronic cellular infiltration and minimal thickening of the glandular epithelium. Such an alteration is to be found in association with hepatitis, regional enteritis, jejunal diverticulosis, ulcerative colitis, kwashiorkor, pernicious anaemia, after partial gastrectomy and after neomycin therapy. Similar changes may be found in coeliac disease and cannot be used to substantiate the diagnosis. The mucosal biopsies are normal in disaccharide deficiency, iron-deficiency anaemia, peptic ulcer disease and pancreatic disease. Villous abnormalities have been described in association with certain skin diseases such as eczema and psoriasis. These are usually non-specific changes, but occasionally a severe atrophy is present which is indistinguishable from coeliac disease.

The biopsy specimen can be stained with special histochemical stains to show various intracellular enzymes such as alkaline phosphatase. The biopsy sample can be frozen to −20°C and used for enzyme estimation. This has been used in the diagnosis of disaccharide deficiency states.

Electron microscopy has been used to identify subtle changes in the mucosa and to search for bacteria in Whipple's disease.

References

Prout BJ. A rapid method of obtaining a jejunal biopsy using a Crosby capsule and gastrointestinal fibrescope. *Gut* 1974; **15**: 571–2

Evans N, Farrow LJ, Harding A, Stewart JS. New techniques for speeding small intestinal biopsy. *Gut* 1970; **11**: 88–9

Rachmilewitz D, Saunders DR. An improvement in the ease of passing a hydraulic biopsy tube. *Gastroenterology* 1975; **49**: 571–2

Crosby WH, Kugler HW. Intraluminal biopsy of the small intestine. *Am J Dig Dis* 1975; **2**: 236–41

Bradborg LL, Rybin GE, Quinton WE. A multipurpose instrument for suction biopsy of the oesophagus, stomach, small bowel and colon. *Gastroenterology* 1959; **37**: 1–16

Flick AL, Quinton WE, Rubin CE. A personal hydraulic biopsy tube for multiple sampling at any level of the gastrointestinal tract. *Gastroenterology* 1961; **40**: 120–6

Owen RL, Brandborg LL. Mucosal histopathology of malabsorption. *Clin Gastroenterol* 1983; **12**: 575–90

Taylor RH, Waterman S. Single intubation test for investigation of malabsorption and diarrhoea. *Gut* 1983; **24**: 680–2

Linscheer WG, Abele JE. A new directable small bowel biopsy device. *Gastroenterology* 1976; **71**: 575–6

Salter RH, Girdwood TG. Peroral jejunal biopsy with Watson capsule and Scott–Harden duodenal intubation tube. *Lancet* 1983; **2**: 1460

RADIOLOGY (Figures 12 and 13)

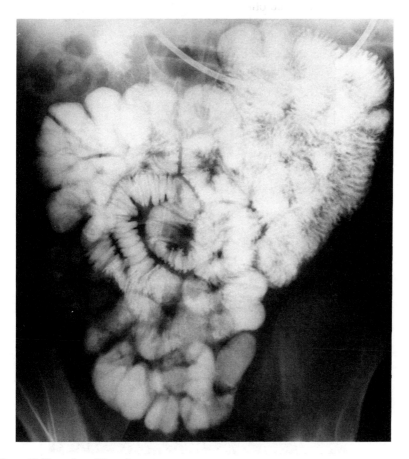

Figure 12 Normal small bowel enema

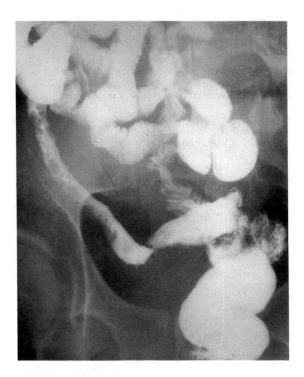

Figure 13(a) Small bowel enema showing terminal ileal Crohn's disease

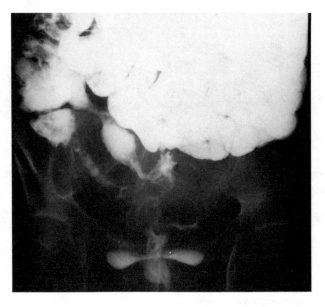

Figure 13(b) Same patient as (a), showing ileo-colo-vesical fistula with barium in the bladder

Though the small intestine can be studied after radiological examination of the stomach has been completed, during the course of a *barium follow-through series* there is unpredictable emptying of the stomach, there may be irregular and excessive filling of the intestine and the barium-filled stomach may obscure parts of the intestine. These difficulties are obviated by the use of the Scott–Harden tube which enables the duodenum to be filled rapidly by a known volume of barium. In this manner a *small bowel enema* is performed using small volumes of relatively dilute barium.

The normal small intestinal mucosa demonstrates a feathery pattern. In coeliac disease there is slowing of the transit time, the bowel lumen is dilated, intestinal folds appear thickened, and there is 'stacking' and clumping of the barium. Barium sulphate tends to flocculate in the presence of steatorrhoea, whether this is the consequence of intestinal or hepatic or pancreatic disease. The use of non-flocculating barium suspensions enables the radiologist to study the intestinal mucosa in the presence of steatorrhoea, and it is of help in the diagnosis of Crohn's disease, strictures, diverticula and blind loops. The terminal ileum may be better outlined by a barium enema than by small bowel follow-through techniques.

Angiographic techniques are available and there is a selective technique in which the catheter is introduced into either the coeliac, or superior or inferior mesenteric artery. It is possible to demonstrate vascular lesions involving the major vessels supplying the gastrointestinal tract. In this way it is possible to demonstrate neoplastic disease of the bowel as well as the site of gastrointestinal bleeding.

Lymphangiography has proved of value in the diagnosis of retroperitoneal lesions and in the demonstration of abnormal intestinal lymphatics such as are found in intestinal lymphangiectasia.

Retrograde ileography via a colonoscopically placed catheter has been described, but not fully evaluated.

Reference

Whorwell PJ, Maxton DG, Martin DL. Post-colonoscopic retrograde ileography. *Lancet* 1988; 1: 738–9

RADIO-ISOTOPE STUDIES

A number of methods have been used but none has yet entered universal practice.

^{67}Gallium scanning

^{67}Gallium citrate localizes in tumours and inflammatory areas. It can be used to delineate ulcerative colitis and also abdominal abscesses in Crohn's disease and other conditions, though uncomplicated Crohn's disease usually yields negative scans.

The technique is simple but ultrasonography and digestive endoscopy probably yield the same information.

Labelled leukocytes

^{111}Indium-autologous leukocytes may be very helpful in assessing the extent of inflammatory bowel disease, but positive abdominal scanning does not establish the diagnosis without other corroborative evidence. The actual faecal excretion of ^{111}indium may help in analysis too. This is $<1\%$ in irritable bowel syndrome and $<1.6\%$ in organic disease excluding ulcerative colitis and Crohn's disease, but $3.6-13.1\%$ in severe inflammatory bowel disease. The method is tedious and expensive, so an alternative using ^{99m}technetium complexed with hexamethylpropylene-amineoxime, and incorporated into leukocytes before scanning, could prove a more practical alternative.

Other technetium scans

^{99m}Technetium-labelled sucralfate has been stated to give good localisation of active inflammatory bowel disease, though the procedure has proved erratic in other hands. ^{99m}Technetium-bran scanning may demonstrate abnormal ileal retention in irritable bowel syndrome. This can be helpful in giving a positive confirmation in diagnosis of this very common condition, but false negatives are not uncommon.

References

Hanser MF, Alderson PO. Gallium-67 imaging in abdominal disease. *Semin Nucl Med* 1982; **8**: 251–70

Holdstock G, Ligorria JE, Krawitt EL. Gallium-67 scanning in patients with Crohn's disease: An aid to the diagnosis of abdominal abscess. *Br J Surg* 1982; **69**: 277–8

Rheingold OJ, Tedesco FJ, Block FE, Maldonado A, Miale A Jr. [^{67}Ga] citrate scintiscanning in active inflammatory bowel disease. *Dig Dis Sci* 1979; **24**: 363–8

Saverymuttu SH, Peters AM, Lavender JP, Hodgson HJ, Chadwick VS. ^{111}Indium autologous leukocytes in inflammatory bowel disease. *Gut* 1983; **24**: 293–9

Saverymuttu SH, Lavender JP, Hodgson HJF, Chadwick VS. Assessment of disease activity in inflammatory bowel disease: a new approach using ^{111}indium in granulocyte scanning. *Br Med J* 1983; **287**: 1751–3

Peters AM, Osman S, Henderson BL, Kelly JD, Danpure HJ, Hawker RJ, Hodgson HJ,

Neirinckx RD. Clinical experience with ^{99m}Tc-hexamethylpropylene- amineoxime for labelling leukocytes and imaging inflammation. *Lancet* 1986; **25**: 946 – 9

Dawson DJ, Khan AN, Miller V, Ratcliffe JF, Shreeve DR. Detection of inflammatory bowel disease in adults and children: evaluation of a new isotopic technique. *Br J Med* 1985; **291**: 1227 – 30

Trotman IF, Price CC. Bloated irritable bowel syndrome defined by dynamic ^{99m}Tc bran scan. *Lancet* 1986; 364 – 7

PROTEIN LOSS

Excessive protein loss into the gastrointestinal tract is a non-specific feature in a number of diseases directly or indirectly affecting the gastrointestinal tract. The loss of protein may present as oedema and hypoalbuminaemia, the clinical syndrome being known as protein-losing gastroenteropathy. Thus tests for the loss of protein into the bowel are important in the clinical investigation of a patient with unexplained hypoalbuminaemia and oedema, particularly when associated with gastrointestinal symptoms.

The quantitative evaluation of enteric protein loss has been attempted either using macromolecular substances with radioactive labels such as [131]iodine, or the inert polyvinylpyrolidine (PVP). However, the development of techniques for quantitating actual protein loss, and of labelling the patient's own albumin *in vivo* represent an improvement.

[51]Chromic chloride

After an injection of [51]chromic chloride most of the label attaches to serum albumin, though some binds to red cells and some is excreted unchanged in the urine.

Method

One hundred microcuries of [51]chromic chloride suspended in saline is injected intravenously. Stools are collected for 5 days, homogenized and made up to a constant volume such as 500 ml. The total radioactivity in the stool collection is counted.

Interpretation

Normal subjects excrete less than 1% of the injected radioactivity in stool. Patients with enteric protein loss lose more than 1% and values of up to 40% may be seen. This method obviates the problem of requiring freshly labelled exogenous albumin in the ^{51}Cr-labelled albumin method. It gives good results in practice.

Radio-iodinated serum protein

^{131}I- or ^{125}I-labelled albumin can be used as the test substance. The method cannot be used for accurate quantitation of intestinal protein loss because of the rapid reabsorption of the radio-iodide label after catabolism of the protein in the gut, and also because of the secretion of the labelled iodine in salivary and gastric secretions. The use of an oral ion exchange resin (Amberlite) which is given in conjunction with the intravenous iodinated albumin has not overcome these difficulties.

Method

Preparations of radio-iodinated serum albumin which may be used to determine volume and cardiac output are not suitable for measuring intestinal protein loss; it is necessary to purchase commercial materials which are specially prepared for this purpose. Each new preparation of iodinated albumin must be tested in a control subject with normal protein metabolism.

The patient is given 0.5 ml aqueous iodine solution orally four times a day from the day before the test until the completion of the study. Sixty microcuries of iodinated albumin are injected intravenously and blood samples are collected without a tourniquet 10–20 min later and then daily for 21 days. Quantitative 24-hour urine samples are obtained throughout the study. All stools are collected and assayed for radioactivity. The serum albumin concentration is determined weekly.

The data may be analysed in a variety of ways. Isotope dilution measurements are made of the plasma volume and the intravascular and total albumin pools. The albumin turnover (g/day) is calculated and this equals the albumin synthetic rate if the patient is in a steady state. In protein-losing enteropathies the increased intestinal loss is reflected in an increased disappearance of plasma radioactivity, and faecal radioactivity is significantly elevated above normal values. Quantitative evaluation is not possible except where abnormal protein loss is restricted to the stomach when a quantitative study is possible using gastric suction.

This method is complex for routine use, but it provides much information which is of value for research purposes.

Other methods

Tests using ^{59}Fe-labelled dextran and ^{67}Cu-labelled caeruloplasmin give good results. ^{59}Fe-labelled dextran found in stools in the 4 days after an i.v. injection of 0.1–0.2 mcCi/kg is normally less than 1%, and this isotope is attractive because it is relatively cheap and it is stable.

Simultaneous administration of ^{131}I-labelled albumin and ^{125}I-labelled IgG followed by differential faecal counting has been advocated as an index of small bowel activity in Crohn's disease, where the ratio of ^{125}I:^{131}I is >1.60.

Alpha$_1$-antitrypsin clearance

Gastrointestinal loss of plasma proteins may also conveniently be measured by estimation of the faecal clearances of the endogenous marker alpha$_1$-antitrypsin, which forms the main alpha$_1$-globulin, with a serum level of 1.9–5.0 g/l. In protein loss the stool level is higher, though the serum concentration is still usually within the normal range. A more sophisticated variant actually calculates alpha$_1$-antitrypsin clearance over 10 days, but has the serious practical drawback of prolonged stool collection.

Indications

The tests are of value in any patient with oedema and low serum albumin concentrations in whom the cause of the hypoalbuminaemia is not apparent. Protein loss into the bowel has been recorded in congestive cardiac failure, giant rugal hypertrophy of the stomach, gastric cancer, intestinal lymphangiectasia, regional enteritis, Whipple's disease, ulcerative colitis and allergic states involving the gastrointestinal tract.

References

Walker-Smith JA, Skyring AP, Mistilis GP. Use of ^{51}CrCl$_3$ in the diagnosis of protein-losing enteropathy. *Gut* 1967; **8**: 166–8

Rubini ME, Sheahy TW. Exudative enteropathy. A comparative study of ^{51}CrCl$_3$ and ^{131}I-PVP. *J Lab Clin Med* 1961; **58**: 892–901

Waldman TA, Wocher RD, Strober W. The role of the gastrointestinal tract in plasma protein-metabolism studies with ^{51}Cr-albumin. *Am J Med* 1969; **46**: 275–85

Kerr RM, Dubois JJ, Holt PR. Use of the ^{125}I- and ^{51}Cr-labelled albumin for the measurement of gastrointestinal and total albumin catabolism. *J Clin Invest* 1967; **46**: 2064–82

Jarnum S, Westergaard H, Yssing M, Jensen H. Quantitation of gastrointestinal protein loss by means of ^{59}Fe-labelled iron dextran. *Gastroenterology* 1968; **55**: 229–41

Jarnum S, Jensen KB. Faecal radioiodine excretion following iv injection of ^{131}I-albumin and ^{125}I-immunoglobulin G in chronic inflammatory bowel disease. *Gastroenterology* 1975; **68**:

1433–44

Crossley JR, Elliott RB. Simple method of diagnosing protein-loss enteropathies. *Br Med J* 1977; **1**: 428–9

Florent C, L'Hirondel C, Desmazures C, Aymes C, Bernier JJ. Intestinal clearance of 1-antitrypsin: a sensitive method for the detection of protein-losing enteropathy. *Gastroenterology* 1981; **81**: 777–80

INTESTINAL BACTERIA

Under normal conditions the small bowel contains only low concentrations of micro-organisms. Bacterial overgrowth occurs in a number of disease states and the assessment of intestinal bacteria is of great value. Methods for determining the extent of bacterial proliferation in the bowel are:

(1)   culture after intubation and aspiration of small bowel contents;
(2)   biopsy of intestinal mucosa;
(3) ^{14}C-labelled glycocholate and ^{14}C-xylose breath tests;
(4)   urinary indican measurement;
(5)   breath hydrogen assay.

Intubation

The small bowel bacterial flora can be directly identified and quantitated by intubation techniques. Intestinal bacteria may be obtained at operation by needle aspiration of the bowel or by a special stainless-steel capsule which has a hollow connection at the proximal end linking to radio-opaque tubing. Suction to the tubing displaces the cap with aspiration of the intestinal contents. The capsule is self-sealing once suction has been discontinued. These methods are no more accurate than using a simple sterilized disposable double-lumen radio-opaque tube.

Method

The intestine is intubated after an overnight fast. The patient, who must not be taking antibiotic therapy, has an alkaline gargle before swallowing the tube. The tube is screened into the desired position, aspirates being taken from the mid-jejunum or any known diseased area. The tube is withdrawn once samples have been obtained. The aspirated samples are delivered to the laboratory as rapidly as possible and plated for aerobic and anaerobic culture. A quantitative and qualitative determination is made of the bacterial population. Strict attention to culture conditions is necessary for demonstration of obligatory anaerobes. Simultaneous culture of saliva is advisable to identify non-significant contaminants.

Interpretation

Normally the jejunum is sterile or bacterial counts are less than $10^3 - 10^5$ per ml, the organisms being mainly of the oropharyngeal type. Counts of more than 10^5 organisms per ml indicate bacterial overgrowth, the organisms being mainly strains of *Escherichia coli* and *Bacteroides*.

Indications

An assessment of intestinal bacterial growth is of value in two ways. The procedure can be used to decide whether steatorrhoea, vitamin B_{12} deficiency or protein malnutrition is the result of bacterial overgrowth in the small bowel. This could be the consequence of intestinal stasis from strictures, fistulas, diverticula or abnormalities of motility. On the other hand it is sometimes of value to know whether there is bacterial overgrowth in patients with strictures, diverticula or abnormal motility of the small intestine.

^{14}C-labelled glycocholic acid breath test

This is based on the ability of many, but not all, intestinal bacteria to deconjugate bile acids. This normally only occurs to any extent in the colon. If there is colonization of the upper small bowel deconjugation results in the absorption of ^{14}C-labelled glycine. This is completely metabolized, producing $^{14}CO_2$ which is measured in the breath.

Method

The patient is fasted overnight. Five microcuries of ^{14}C-glycine-glycocholic acid is given by mouth and the patient is then allowed to eat normally. Before, and at hourly intervals for 7 hours after the isotope has been administered, breath is collected by bubbling through a solution containing 1 mmol hyamine hydroxide with thymolphthalein indicator until the blue colour disappears.

The radioactivity in each sample is measured by liquid scintillation counting.

Interpretation

Results are expressed as % dose of ^{14}C excreted/mmol CO_2 trapped, corrected for body weight. In normal subjects values in each of the first 3 hours are below 0.1%, and no value throughout the test exceeds 0.3%.

In upper small bowel bacterial overgrowth values from 2 hours onwards are raised, with maximal values at 3–5 hours. In cholangitis peak values are seen at 1–2 hours. In intestinal hurry normal colonic bacteria may give late positive results. An internal bile fistula usually invalidates the test.

Unfortunately this test has not fulfilled its early promise of replacing the need for small bowel intubation and direct culture.

Similarly the ^{14}C-xylose test is not widely used.

Urinary indican

In patients with excessive bacterial growth in the small intestine there is an increase in the excretion of indican (indoxyl sulphate) in the urine. The indoles are produced by bacterial activity, particularly *Escherichia coli* and *Bacteroides*, or by tryptophan in the diet.

With the patient on a normal diet a 24-hour urine collection is made into a bottle containing a few millilitres of either chloroform or thymol.

The normal output of indican in the urine is 48 ±20 mg/24 hours. Values above 80 mg/24 hours are abnormal. Slight elevations are present in a variety of diseases such as coeliac disease without necessarily indicating significant bacterial overgrowth. Values above 100 mg/24 hours imply profuse bacterial proliferation, but the test is too erratic in performance to be very useful.

Breath hydrogen

Bacterial colonisation of the small intestine leads to an increase in breath hydrogen to more than 20 ppm after a 50 g glucose load by mouth. Unfortunately the values may be spuriously raised in cigarette smokers, after dietary carbohydrate intake and in intestinal hurry and irritable bowel syndrome; and may be reduced by exercise and hyperventilation. The test requires very careful standardisation to be useful, despite the deceptive ease with which breath hydrogen can be monitored by automatic machines.

Biopsy

Endoscopic forceps biopsy and simultaneous intestinal aspiration followed by microscopy and culture can be very helpful in diagnosis of giardiasis, and perhaps also in *Campylobacter*-like infections.

References

Goka AKJ, Rolston DDK, Mathan VI, Farthing MJG. Diagnosis of giardiasis by specific IgM antibody enzyme-linked immunosorbent assay. *Lancet* 1986; **2**: 184 – 6

Attwood SEA, Mealy K, Cafferkey MT, *et al.* Yersinia infection and acute abdominal pain. *Lancet* 1987; **1**: 529 – 33

Watson WS, Mckenzie I, Holden RI, Craig L, Sleight JD, Crean GP. An evaluation of the ^{14}C-glycocholic acid breath test in the diagnosis of bacterial colonisation of the jejunum. *Scottish Med J* 1980; **25**: 25 – 32

James OFW, Agnew JE, Bouchier IAD. Assessment of the ^{14}C-glycocholic acid breath test. *Br Med J* 1973; **3**: 191 – 5

Curzon G, Walsh J. A method for the determining of urinary indican. *Clin Chem Acta* 1962; **7**: 657 – 63

King CE, Toskes PP. Small intestinal bacterial overgrowth. *Gastroenterology* 1979; **76**: 1035 – 55 (review)

Mackowiak PA. The normal microbial flora. *N Engl J Med* 1982, **307**: 83 – 93

Hamilton I, Wolsey BW, Cobden I, Cooke EM, Shoesmith JG, Axon ATR. Simultaneous culture of saliva and jejunal aspirate in the investigation of small bowel bacterial overgrowth. *Gut* 1982; **23**: 847 – 53

Thompson DG, Binfield P, De Belder A, O'Brien J, Warren S, Wilson M. Extra-intestinal influences on exhaled breath hydrogen measurements during the investigation of gastrointestinal disease. *Gut* 1985; **26**: 1349 – 52

Gordts B, Hemelhof W, Retore P, Rahman M, Cadranel S, Butzler JP. Routine culture of *giardia lamblia* trophozoites from human duodenal aspirates. *Lancet* 1984; **2**: 137

Levitt MD, Hirsch P, Fetzer CA, Sheaman M, Levine AS. H_2 excretion after ingestion of complex carbohydrates. *Gastroenterology* 1987; **92**: 383 – 9

INTESTINAL MOTILITY

The measurement and monitoring of intestinal motility are undertaken with difficulty in man and are rarely necessary in the clinical evaluation of a patient with gastrointestinal symptoms. Small intestinal motility is measured most conveniently by radiology but the results are very variable. Barium sulphate may well stimulate bowel activity and its rate of passage is not an index of the transit time for ordinary meals. Transit time is claimed to be more rapid when the patient is in the right lateral recumbent position and slower when there are faeces in the colon. It usually takes 60 – 90 min for barium to reach the colon. There is reduced intestinal motility when there is steatorrhoea. On the other hand patients with lactose intolerance have intestinal hurry and this may be demonstrated by the ingestion of a test meal containing 100 g micro-opaque barium sulphate suspension mixed with 25 g lactose.

The radiological assessment of intestinal motility is often sufficient for clinical purposes.

Markers

Markers are used during studies on the gastrointestinal tract:

(1)   Non-absorbable markers are incorporated into test solutions to be in-fused during perfusion studies. The dilution or concentration of the marker in samples of the perfusion fluid theoretically measures the flow rates and volumes of the intestinal contents at the site of study. Polyethylene glycol (PEG) and phenol red are the two markers of most value for perfusion studies. Marker perfusion techniques are used primarily during physiological studies of intestinal absorption. Radio-opaque solid markers with radiology of patient and/or stools can be used to assess transit.

(2)   Markers have also been used to assess or fix the duration of a stool collection. However, this is seldom required in clinical practice and during a 3- or 5-day collection of faeces for fat excretion no markers are used. More precise timing may be required during metabolic balance studies.

Method

Chromium sesquioxide

A capsule containing 0.5 g chromium sesquioxide is taken three times a day with the meals and the amount of marker in grams recovered in the faeces is divided by 1.5 to give the number of days represented by the collection. A method described by Clarkson enables a measurement to be made within 1 hour; the homogenized faeces are wet-digested with nitric and perchloric acids and the optical density of the dichromate is measured in a colorimeter.

Carmine No. 40

This is a red, non-absorbable dye which is readily recognized in the stool. The dye is administered in capsules (usually 3 – 4 g) at varying intervals to in-dicate different periods represented by the stool collection. This method suf-fers from erratic mixing of the dye and the difficulties of interpretation when the patient is constipated. Charcoal may be used in a similar way.

   Markers are used clinically to detect whether an abdominal fistula is a faecal fistula. Carmine and charcoal are useful in this respect.

Radiotelemetry and manometry

Specialized units have developed ways of estimating pressures and both electrical and motor activity in the stomach and small intestine. This has improved understanding of physiology, and led to the definition of a discrete form of functional bowel disease (chronic idiopathic intestinal pseudo-obstruction). However, analysis of results is complicated by normal variability, and the effects of stress and the menstrual cycle, so the technique does not have general applicability.

References

Clarkson EM. A rapid method for the determination of chromium sesquioxide in faecal homogenates. *Clin Chem Acta* 1966; **16**: 571–2

Stanghellini V, Camilleri M, Malagelada J-R. Chronic idiopathic intestinal pseudo-obstruction (CIIP): Clinical and intestinal manometric findings. *Gut* 1987; **28**: 5–12

Kerlin P, Phillips S. Variability of motility of the ileum and jejunum in healthy humans. *Gastroenterology* 1982; **82**: 694–700

Thompson DG, Wingate DL, Archer L, Benson MJ, Green WJ, Hardy RJ. Normal patterns of human upper small bowel activity recorded by prolonged radiotelemetry. *Gut* 1980; **21**: 500–6

Wald A, Van Thiel DH, Hoechstetter L. Gastrointestinal transit the effect of the menstrual cycle. *Gastroenterology* 1981; **80**: 994–8

McCrae S, Younger K, Thompson DG, Wingate DL. Sustained mental stress alters human jejunal motor activity. *Gut* 1982; **23**: 404–9

Connel AM. Motility and its disturbances. *Clin Gastroenterol* 1982; **11**: 437–686

CROHN'S DISEASE

This is often difficult to diagnose and a number of helpful tests are available:

Excision biopsy of involved sites

Full thickness of inflammation, deep ulcers and granulomas are diagnostic features. Local lymph nodes may also contain granulomas.

Barium radiology

Internal fistulas between loops of small bowel and skin lesions (diseased areas separated by normal bowel) are the most helpful findings, though a host of other abnormalilities occur.

Rectal biopsies and upper gastrointestinal biopsies

Sometimes diagnostic features are seen, but often non-specific changes can be identified which support a diagnosis of organic disease.

Skin testing with tuberculin, dinitrochlorbenzene (DNCB) and the Kveim test

The Mantoux test is negative in most patients with active Crohn's disease, even if they have been immunized against tuberculosis. Anergy to DNCB (i.e. no reaction after skin injection) occurs in 70%, compared with 9% of controls. The Kveim test is a cutaneous injection of a prepared extract of spleen from diseased patients which provokes a granulomatous reaction, identified by histology at 6 weeks. It is positive in about half the patients with Crohn's disease.

Other tests

Colonoscopy may be able to visualize directly the terminal ileum or involved large bowel. The SeHCAT and Schilling tests are abnormal in terminal ileitis. Urinary oxalate excretion and faecal fat excretion are often increased. Granulocytes labelled with ^{67}gallium citrate and ^{111}indium may locate diseased areas (both active regional enteritis and abscesses). Ultrasonography can be helpful in diagnosis. T- and B-lymphocyte functions are usually depressed, but this is variable.

Investigations for monitoring progress

Because of the variability and chronicity of Crohn's disease, attempts have been made to establish investigations which might correlate with disease activity. Serial measurements of serum seromucoids and lysozyme, C-reactive protein, plasma viscosity, and regular barium radiology have not proved very useful in practice.

A simple index of Crohn's disease activity based on history and physical examination has been found satisfactory. This uses a scoring system based on:

general wellbeing (0 = very well, 4 = terrible)
abdominal pain (0 = rare, 3 = severe)
daily numberof liquid stools
abdominal mass (0 = absent, 3 = definite + tender)
complications, e.g. arthralgia, aphthous ulcers (score 1 each).

A patient who is perfectly well scores 0, and a patient who is in severe relapse, scores more than 10.

In addition, serial ultrasonography and serial weighing in patients not on steroids, give some helpful objective data. The ESR and a full blood count including platelets (raised in active disease) are practical simple objective yardsticks.

References

Holt G, Samuel E. Grey scale ultrasound in Crohn's disease. *Gut* 1979; **20**: 59–595

Harvey RF, Bradshaw IM. A simple index of Crohn's disease activity. *Lancet* 1980; **i**: 514

Van Hees PAM, Van Elteren PH, Van Lier HJJ, Van Tongeren JHM. An index of inflammatory activity in patients with Crohn's disease. *Gut* 1980; **21**: 279–86

Andre C, Descos L, Landais P, Fermanian J. Assessment of appropriate laboratory measurement to supplement the Crohn's disease activity index. *Gut* 1981; **22**: 571–4

Brignola C, Campieri M, Bazzochi G, Farruggia P, Tragone A, Lan Franch EA. A laboratory index for predicting relapse in asymptomatic patients with Crohn's disease. *Gastroenterology* 1986; **91**: 1490–4

Miller A, Green M, Robinson D. Simple rule for calculating normal erythrocyte sedimentation rate. *Br Med J* 1983; **286**: 266

Harries AD, Fitzsimons E, Fifield R, Dew MJ, Rhodes J. Platelet count: a simple measure of activity in Crohn's disease. *Br Med J* 1983; **286**: 1476

Admans H, Whorwell PJ, Wright R, Phil D. Diagnosis of Crohn's disease. *Dig Dis Sci* 1980; **25**: 911–15

Chadwick VS. Diagnosis and medical management of Crohn's disease. *Br J Hosp Med* 1982; 472–80

METABOLIC DISORDERS

Gastrointestinal symptoms such as pain, diarrhoea and constipation may be the most prominent features of certain metabolic disorders. During the investigation of a patient with abdominal pain, it may be helpful to determine the serum calcium (elevated in hyperparathyroidism) and to note whether the serum is lactescent (in certain forms of hyperlipidaemia). Abdominal pain may be an early feature of diabetic ketosis and a manifestation of a haemolytic crisis as in sickle cell anaemia. Hypothyroidism may present with constipation, and diarrhoea can be prominent in pellagra.

CARCINOID SYNDROME

Patients with hepatic metastases from a primary carcinoid tumour in the gut may present with a syndrome of intermittent diarrhoea, flushing, asthma and a pellagrinous rash. Occasionally diarrhoea dominates the clinical picture. Diagnostic tests are based on the knowledge that these tumours contain a high concentration of 5-hydroxytryptamine (5-HT, serotonin) which is converted to 5-hydroxyindoleacetic acid (5-HIAA) and excreted in excess in the urine.

Screening test

A screening test for 5-HIAA is available based on the reaction of 5-HIAA with 1-nitrose-2-naphthol.

Method

0.2 ml urine, 0.5 ml nitrosonaphthol reagent (1% nitrosonaphthol in 100% ethanol), 0.5 ml freshly prepared nitrous acid reagent (0.2 ml of 2.5% sodium nitrate and 2.5 ml mol/l sulphuric acid) and 0.8 ml distilled water are mixed together in a test tube and allowed to stand at room temperature for 10–15 min. Five millilitres ethylene dichloride is added and the layers allowed to separate. If turbidity occurs the tube is centrifuged.

Interpretation

A positive test is indicated by a purple colour in the top layer and indicates an excess of urinary 5-HIAA. In normal urine there is no purple colour or occasionally a light yellow appearance.

Three successive early morning samples should be tested. The patient should not be taking bananas which contain large amounts of 5-HT, or mephenesin, acetanilide or phenothiazine derivatives, all of which interfere with the colour reaction.

Twenty-four hour urinary excretion

The urine is collected into a bottle containing 25 ml glacial acetic acid to preserve the 5-HIAA, which is measured in the laboratory. Normally less than 9 mg 5-HIAA are excreted in 24 hours. In the carcinoid syndrome values are 40–873 mg/24 hours. A moderate increase of urinary 5-HIAA, 9–20 mg/24 hours has been reported in untreated adult coelic disease, tropical sprue and Whipple's disease.

Platelet serotonin

Fasting blood is collected into a heparin tube. The normal platelet serotonin content is less than 0.4 mcg/mg protein. In the carcinoid syndrome values are between 0.64 – 3.54 mcg/mg protein.

PHAEOCHROMOCYTOMA

Occasionally the possibility is raised that diarrhoea is due to the presence of a phaeochromocytoma. Diagnosis of this tumour is based on measurement of the 24-hour excretion of urinary catecholamines and metabolites, which are elevated in phaeochromocytoma. The excretion of these substances is occasionally paroxysmal. Therapy with methyldopa is stopped for 3 days before the test because this drug can give false-positive tests. For 2 days before the test the patient should not receive caffeine products, red plums, tomatoes or food with vanilla essence such as ice cream.

The 24-hour urinary output is collected into a bottle containing 12 ml concentrated hydrochloric acid. The urine may be tested for 3-methoxy-4-hydroxymandelic acid (vanilyl mandelic acid, VMA), which is a simple test, or for the output of metadrenaline or of catecholamines. Normally less than 6.5 mg/24 hours VMA is excreted, less than 1.3 mg/24 hours metadrenaline and less than 20 mcg adrenaline/24 hours and 8 mcg noradrenaline/24 hours.

References

Asmark E, Knutsson F, Thoren L. Phaeochromocytoma: diagnostic features. *Acta Med Scand* 1967; **182**: 673 – 80

PORPHYRIA

Acute abdominal pain may be a prominent feature in various forms of porphyria including acute intermittent porphyria and variegate porphyria.

Urinary porphyrins

The Watson – Schwartz test for porphobilinogen is a widely used screening test. Equal volumes of urine and Ehrlich's reagent are mixed in a test tube and allowed to stand for 3 min. Two volumes saturated sodium acetate solution are added. A few millilitres of chloroform are added after a few minutes and the test tube shaken. Porphobilinogen forms a reddish compound which is insoluble in chloroform. Extraction into an amyl alcohol/benzyl alcohol mixture (3:1, v/v) is said to increase the accuracy of the test. This test is liable to false-positive and false-negative reactions, and it has been suggested that the screening test should always be confirmed by quantitative determinations. The normal 24-hour excretion of porphobilinogen is not more than 2.0 mg, with a mean of 1.5 mg. The normal excretion of delta-aminolaevulinic acid is up to 4.5 mg/24 hours with a mean of 2.5 mg/24 hours.

Faecal porphyrins

An increased excretion of coproporphyrins and protoporphyrins may be the only detectable biochemical abnormality in some forms of porphyria, such as variegate porphyria and hereditary coproporphyria. A useful screening test is to mix 1 ml ether, 1 ml glacial acetic acid and 1 ml amyl alcohol in a test tube and add a small amount of crushed faeces. The faecal extract is exposed to ultraviolet light. An excess of porphyrins is indicated by a red fluorescene. Chlorophyll derivatives give fluorescence as well; although porphyrins can be extracted with dilute hydrochloric acid it is advisable to check a positive screening test by quantitative determination.

The upper limit of the normal total faecal porphyrins is between 100–150 mcg/g dry weight of stool. The normal coproporphyrin excretion is 8 mcg/g dry weight of stool and for protoporphyrin is 21 mcg/g dry weight of stool.

LEAD INTOXICATION

Abdominal pain may be a prominent feature of lead poisoning. Nowadays measurement of serum lead is a readily available investigation which is probably the best test. Screening tests of value include the demonstration of an excess urinary excretion of coproporphyrin III and delta-aminolaevulinic acid. A few ml of urine are acidified with acetic acid, mixed with an equal volume of ether and exposed to ultraviolet light. A positive test is given by a red fluorescence of the ether layer. Another useful screening test is the demonstration of basophilic stippling of the erythrocytes. Quantitative estimations of the excretion of lead in the urine may be undertaken, and 0.2 mg/l is generally considered to be a significant concentration.

IMMUNOLOGY

This has had less impact on diagnosis than might have been expected. The

Widal test remains a useful tool in typhoid, but is often difficult to interpret after immunization. Specific serum antigen assay shows promise. *Lymphocyte function* and the absolute *numbers of B- and T-lymphocytes* circulating in the blood can be shown to be disturbed in various bowel diseases. Typing the *human leukocyte antigens* may be helpful. Of patients with coeliac disease 80% have HLA-A1 and -B8, and there is an increased frequency of HLA-B5 in Behçet's disease.

In coeliac disease the *immunoglobulin pattern* is characteristic; the serum IgA level is low, normal or mildly raised, with low IgM and IgG levels. After gluten exclusion the IgA level tends to fall and a subsequent rise may indicate poor adherence to diet or lymphoma formation.

Alpha$_1$-Gliadin and *IgA-class reticulin antibodies* appear to be a specific finding in patients with coeliac disease on a normal diet and their relatives. IgG-class reticulin antibodies are found both in coeliac disease and inflammatory bowel disease.

References

Mak M, Hallstrom O, Vesikari T, *et al.* Evaluation of serum IgA – class reticulin antibody. Test for the detection of childhood coeliac disease. *J Paediatr* 1984; 901 – 5

Cacciari E, Salardi S, Volta U *et al.* Can antigliadin antibody detect symptomless coeliac disease in children with short stature? *Lancet* 1985; 1: 1469 – 71

O'Farrelly C, Kelly J, Hekkens W *et al.* Alpha-gliadin antibodies: a serological test for coeliac disease. *Br Med J* 1983; 286: 2007 – 10

Savilahti E, Viander M, Perkkio M, Vainio E, Kalimo K, Reunala T. IgA antigliadin antibodies: a marker of mucosal damage in childhood coeliac disease. *Lancet* 1983; 1: 320 – 22

Sivadasan K, Kurien B, John TJ. Rapid diagnosis of typhoid fever by antigen detection. *Lancet* 1984; 1: 134 – 5

FOOD ALLERGY AND INTOLERANCE

True food allergy is a contentious subject, and many alleged victims are suffering from psychiatric or other functional complaints.

The presence of *classic atopy*, especially with rhinitis and a positive family history, is a helpful clue to true food allergy. Atopy is often associated with *raised serum IgE levels*, which are up to 100 u/ml in normal adults and up to 50 u/ml in normal children.

Jejunal IgE levels are elevated in true food allergy confirmed by blind allergen food challenge skin and prick tests, mean values being four times normal (261 *versus* 68 u/ml).

Histology of the small intestine may show eosinophil or mononuclear cell infiltration, especially after allergen challenge, with degranulation of mast cells also. Immunofluorescence can show deposition of IgE and immune complexes, together with infiltration of cells secreting IgA and other immunoglobulins.

Double blind challenge with suspected food allergens can provide objective evidence to support or refute diagnosis, but is very laborious and requires in-patient supervision to be effective. It may be reserved for patients whose symptoms improve or disappear with an open hypo-allergenic diet for a week (e.g. the water, lamb, rice and pears regime).

References

Belut D, Moneret-Vautrin DA, Nicholas JP, Grilliat JP. IgE levels in intestinal disease. *J Dig Dis Sci* 1980; **25**: 323-32

Pearson DJ, Rix KJB, Bentley SJ. Food allergy: How much in the mind? A clinical and psychiatric study of suspected food hypersensitivity. *Lancet* 1983; **1**: 1259-61

Allun-Jones V, McLaughlan P, Shorthouse M, Workman E, Hunter JO. Food intolerance: a major factor in the pathogenesis of irritable bowel syndrome. *Lancet* 1982; **2**: 1115-7

Whorwell PJ, Maxton DG, Martin DF. Post-colonoscopic retrograde ileography. *Lancet* 1988; **1**: 729-738

Aas K. Studies of hypersensitivity to fish-allergological and serological differentiation between various species of fish. *Int Arch Allergy* 1966; **30**: 257

Aas K. The diagnosis of hypersensitivity to ingested foods: reliability of skin prick testing and radioallergosorbent test with different materials. *Clin Allergy* 1978; **8**: 39

Maki M, Hallstrom O, Verronen P *et al*. Reticulin antibody, arthritis and coeliac disease in children. *Lancet* 1988; **1**: 479-80

Dias J, Unsworth DJ, Walker-Smith JA. Antigliadin and antireticulin antibodies in screening for coeliac disease. *Lancet* 1987; **2**: 157-8

Unsworth DJ, Walker-Smith JA, Holborow EJ. Gliadin and reticulin antibodies in childhool coeliac disease. *Lancet* 1983; **1**: 874-5

Colon and rectum

RECTAL EXAMINATION

The importance of the rectal examination cannot be overstressed: it should form part of every complete physical examination. A measure of the importance of the rectal examination is gauged by the fact that about 15% of all large bowel cancers can be felt digitally. It is usually possible to reach further with a finger than can be seen with an anoscope.

Method

Before the examination proper the procedure is explained to the patient who is warned that there may be a desire to defecate. Many patients find this examination both embarrassing and uncomfortable, and they are considerably helped by a sympathetic and understanding attitude on the part of the examiner.

The patient is placed in the left lateral position with the head, trunk and hips well flexed. The buttocks are parted and the anal region inspected. The right index finger, covered by either a glove or a finger cot, is well lubricated and inserted into the anus. It is advisable to use an anaesthetic jelly if a painful lesion such as a thrombosed haemorrhoid or a fissure is suspected, and particular care is exercised in the introduction of the finger, which should be done very slowly. The examiner stands facing the patient's feet and introduces the finger from the posterior anal region. In the case of infants the little finger is used.

There are a number of other positions for the rectal examination. In the left lateral position the left leg can be extended and the right thigh and knee flexed. The dorsal position is useful for a bimanual examination. The knee–chest position is convenient when a prostatic smear is being taken, though many patients find this posture fatiguing and embarrassing and it is not generally recommended.

The tone of the sphincter is noted, the anal muscle felt, and the finger is then introduced to the furthermost extent. It is then swept round in a full circle to examine the whole circumference of the rectum. The sacral curve, the lateral pelvic walls and the pubis are all palpated and the patient is requested to bear down to enable a further inch of the rectum to be palpated.

Particular note is made of the character of the prostate or the cervix and uterus. The female adenexa may be palpated by bimanual examination. After withdrawing the finger the anus is cleaned. The material on the glove is examined and it can be used for microscopy and for testing for occult blood.

Interpretation

Cancer of the rectum will be felt as an indurated ulcerating lesion, a proliferating tumour or a stenosing infiltrative growth.

Rectal polyps can be very soft and may be mistaken for a mass of faeces, and a similar error can be made when palpating an *amoeboma*.

Internal haemorrhoids are not felt unless they are thrombosed, or are so large that they are felt as soft or 'wobbly' excrescences.

Crohn's disease of the rectum causes a nodular and indurated rectal wall.

Secondary deposits on the pelvic floor can be felt through the rectal wall, but care must be taken not to confuse malignant deposits with hard faecal lumps that are being palpated through a rectal valve.

Cancer of the prostate is identified by a 'rock-hard' prostate gland with or without fixation to the anterior rectal wall.

ANOSCOPY (PROCTOSCOPY)

The instrument commonly referred to as a proctoscope is more correctly termed an anal speculum or anoscope. It is used to visualize the anal mucosa and in no way replaces the digital or sigmoidoscopic examination. A variety of instruments is available and an instrument with a good light and a reasonably small diameter should be chosen. There are convenient transparent plastic disposable instruments.

Method

The instrument is warmed in the examiner's hand or in warm water, and it is well lubricated using local anaesthetic jelly if necessary. The patient is reassured and warned about the sensation of defecation. The protoscope is gradually introduced into the anus with the patient in the left lateral position. The examiner stands facing the patient's feet, holding the handle of the proctoscope at the 12 o'clock position. The instrument is slowly inserted by a rotary clockwise movement so that a half circle has been described by the time the instrument is fully inserted. The handle now rests posteriorly between the gluteal folds. The obturator is withdrawn and an examination is made of the mucosa.

Interpretation

Details of mucosal changes in disease are given in the section dealing with the sigmoidoscope. Anoscopic examination is the best means of diagnosing internal haemorrhoids; the patient strains while the instrument is slowly withdrawn and the purplish vessels will be seen to bulge in the left lateral, right posterior and right anterior positions. Secondary, smaller, haemorrhoids may appear between these three primary positions. Other abnormalities to be seen include fissure, fistulas, anal and low rectal cancers, amoebic ulcers and proctitis.

PROCTOSIGMOIDOSCOPY

Proctosigmoidoscopy is an integral part of the examination of the colon. It should always be performed before referring a patient for a barium enema examination. A number of instruments are available. For routine use a rigid 25 cm Welch–Alleyn instrument (or one with a fibreoptic light source) is commonly used. Distal lighting systems have the disadvantage that they are more easily fouled and obscured, but they give superior illumination. A magnifying eyepiece is useful but a telescopic attachment has no particular advantage. Disposable instruments are now widely used.

There is a 60 cm flexible fibreoptic proctosigmoidoscope. This has the advantage that all the rectum and sigmoid colon can be seen: about 75% of large bowel cancers should be visible with this instrument. It is not certain at present whether the routine use of fibreoptic proctosigmoidoscopy will reduce the need for colonoscopy, but flexible instruments are superior to rigid ones for examination of the distal large bowel.

Method for rigid proctosigmoidoscopy

Preparation

The patient is reassured and warned that some discomfort might be felt, which can be alleviated to some extent by deep breathing. There may also be the desire to defecate. Normally no bowel preparation is necessary and the procedure can be undertaken readily on outpatients. Enemas and suppositories have the disadvantage that they alter the natural state of the mucous membrane, washing away secretions and causing hyperaemia, which is an important consideration when the diagnosis of ulcerative colitis is being considered: enemas not only add to the difficulties of making a diagnosis but are potentially dangerous. It is reasonable to give a saline enema if a cancer of the colon is being considered and there is much faecal material. Various disposal enemas are available for outpatient use, but they may all cause mucosal irritation.

Position

The patient may be examined on a surgical table, or an examination couch, or in the hospital bed; in which instance it is helpful to place a fracture board under the mattress to ensure that the patient lies in the correct position. The examination is facilitated by being performed in a semi-darkened room. Two positions are recommended: the left lateral, and the knee-chest. The left lateral is preferred because it is more comfortable for the patient. For the proctosigmoidoscope to be successfully introduced, it is essential that the patient is correctly positioned. The patient is well flexed and lies transversely across the bed with the buttocks positioned at the very edge. The knees are slightly extended. A sandbag or pillow can be placed under the left hip, which is positioned at the edge of the couch. The left shoulder is tucked under the body and the right arm is brought forward. The head rests on a flat pillow. Failure to pass the proctosigmoidoscope fully is frequently the consequence of faulty positioning, particularly when the procedure is performed at the bedside. A soft mattress cause marked twisting of the spine, making it difficult to negotiate the curves in the rectum and lower colon. The position of the examiner is also important; he must be comfortable and relaxed and this is best achieved by either sitting on a low stool or kneeling at the bedside.

The knee-chest position may sometimes be helpful if there is much loose stool and blood, but is much less comfortable for the patient and is not recommended. In this position the knees are well drawn up and the back arched so that there is a distinct lumbar lordosis; the face is turned to one side, the chest and shoulders rest on the couch and the arms drop over the side of the couch.

Multi-purpose tables are available enabling the patient to be tilted into the knee-chest position.

Procedure

Before introducing the instrument the light connections are checked and the proctosigmoidoscope is warmed. It is lubricated and an anaesthetic jelly is used if necessary. A digital examination of the rectum is made and the patient warned that the instrument is about to be introduced.

The obturator is inserted in the proctosigmoidoscope and the instrument held in the right hand. It is introduced into the anus using a rotary movement and the tip is directed forwards for 5 cm in the direction of the umbilicus. The obturator is removed and the eye piece attached. From this point the examination is performed under direct vision. The instrument is now advanced in a backward direction and enters the rectum by following the curve of the sacrum. As the instrument is advanced it may become necessary to separate the mucosal folds by inflating with air, but this is kept to a minimum as it is both uncomfortable for the patient and potentially dangerous. Small pieces of stool usually can be moved out of the way with the end of the instrument; they are sometimes of value in indicating the position of the bowel lumen. Stool which occludes the end of the proctosigmoidoscope may be removed by introducing the obturator, withdrawing the instrument slightly and then removing the obturator. Another way is to displace the stool with a swab which is attached to a swab-holding forceps. Occasionally the forward passage of the instrument is prevented by spasm of the bowel, but if the proctosigmoidoscope is withdrawn slightly and held still for a short while the spasm will disappear and it is possible to proceed with the examination.

The rectal mucosa is smooth and it is easy to see the rectal valves. The rectosigmoid junction is reached 12–15 cm from the anal margin. This is at the level of the sacral promontory and is identified by the change of the mucosa to concentric rugal folds. The rectosigmoid junction is usually sharply angled and may be difficult to traverse: the proctosigmoidoscope is directed anteriorly and to the right but the sharp angling may cause some discomfort. In many examinations it proves impossible to lever the proctosigmoidoscope through the rectosigmoid junction without undue discomfort. The sigmoid colon is not reliably reached without a general anaesthetic. The average penetration is 20 cm in men and 18.5 in women, but it is uncertain how far along the sigmoid colon the instrument passes, and it is probable that a mobile colon is simply displaced forwards. However, about 5 cm of the sigmoid may be seen. The instrument is now slowly withdrawn and the mucosa carefully re-scrutinized and biopsies taken as required. After withdrawal of the instrument the patient is cleaned and any stool adhering to the sigmoidoscope is taken for examination. A full description of the procedure is entered in the patient's notes and this should include the distance to which the proctosigmoidoscope was introduced, the appearance of the mucosa, the presence of blood or mucus and the appearance of the stool, and whether a biopsy was taken and the site.

Method for flexible sigmoidoscopy (Figure 14)

The equipment is conveniently mounted on a small trolley for out-patient use. The patient is prepared by the use of two phosphate enemas given simultaneously, which should normally clear the lower bowel in 30–45 min. The patient is positioned in the left lateral position with the knees flexed, and the lubricated tip of the instrument is advanced into the rectum. It is often necessary to withdraw the instrument a little to obtain a good view of the rectum.

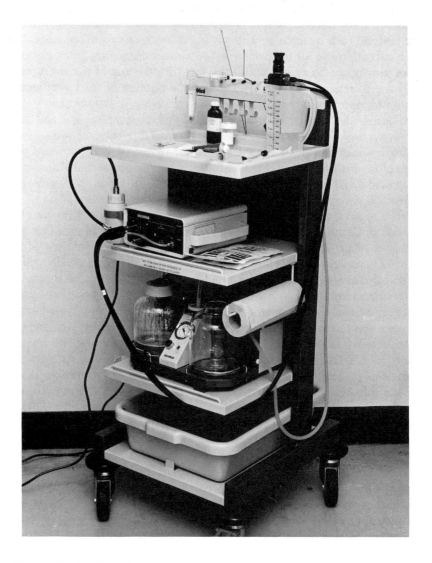

Figure 14 Flexible sigmoidoscopy trolley

It is then possible to advance the instrument under direct vision, steering to keep the lumen in view at all times. With patience and gentle air insufflation it should be possible to view the entire rectum and sigmoid colon with only mild discomfort. Usually the descending colon can be seen also, and it may be possible to reach the splenic flexure or even enter the transverse colon, though unsedated patients do not always tolerate this. When patients are nervous, or where a full examination of the left colon is essential, or where a polypectomy is planned, it is preferable to conduct the procedure in a specialized investigation unit or as a day-ward case. This permits the use of midazolam i.v. to allow a complete passage of the 60 cm instrument to the splenic flexure. Suspect areas can be biopsied with endoscopy forceps: the largest compatible with the instrument are recommended.

Interpretation

When the mucous membrane is examined an overall impression is obtained; particular attention is paid to the vascular pattern and whether there is bleeding, granularity, ulceration and oedema as judged by thickening of the rectal valves.

Normal

The mucous membrane is pink, it is not friable and should not bleed with the gentle passage of the instrument. Undue bleeding during the examination suggests that the mucosa is abnormal. The normal vascular pattern is well visualized and comprises a network of small arterioles and to a lesser extent of venules. The rectal valves are sharp and crescentic in shape. A small amount of mucus may be seen.

Ulcerative colitis and ulcerative proctitis

The appearances vary according to the stage of the disease. In the acute stage the mucosa is reddened, friable, haemorrhagic, and no vascular pattern can be seen. Thickening of the rectal valves almost to the point of obliteration indicates the presence of mucosal oedema. Ulcers are rarely distinguished and when seen appear shallow and irregular. There is nothing specific about these appearances which are to be seen in acute bacillary dysentery, occasionally in amoebic dysentery and in various toxic states. In the subacute and chronic stages of ulcerative colitis the normal vascular pattern is obscured, the mucosa is reddened and granular and bleeds readily when gently stroked by the sigmoidoscope or a swab. It is probable that some degree of mucosal abnormality such as excessive friability remains even with the most chronic and inactive of colonic involvement. proctosigmoidoscopy is of value in distinguishing ulcerative colitis from ulcerative proctitis, in which only the terminal 10–12 cm of bowel is diseased.

Dysentery

The appearance is very similar in bacillary dysentery to that seen in acute ulcerative colitis. The mucosa in amoebic dysentery has small flask-shaped ulcers containing a small bead of pus, but is is otherwise normal. However, the picture is variable and the mucous membrane may be quite reddened and inflammed and at times present a picture not unlike acute ulcerative colitis.

Large bowel malignant disease

About half of all large bowel cancers may be seen with the rigid proctosigmoidoscope. Malignant growths are seen as infiltrating or ulcerating lesions with a varying amount of haemorrhage and necrosis. Other new growths include lobulated pink or red adenomatous polyps and sessile, branching soft villous adenomas. A neoplasm should be suspected if altered or fresh blood is seen in the lumen of the bowel ahead of the proctosigmoidoscope.

Other diseases

Pneumatosis cystoides intestinalis shows as multiple glistening blue-purple submucous cysts.

Granulomatous colitis (Crohn's disease of the colon) is difficult to distinguish from the other forms of colitis, but a nodular 'cobblestone' appearance of the mucosa with discrete ulcers suggests this disease. The rectum is less frequently involved in granulomatous than in ulcerative colitis.

The proctosigmoidoscopic appearnces are not specific in *diverticulitis*; the mucosa may be reddened or normal, and the orifices of the diverticula will be seen with the flexible instrument.

A false impression of the colonic mucosas is obtained when suppositories or enemas are given prior to examination. The mucosa may become reddened and oedematous and appear very abnormal. Difficulties are also found in patients with severe diarrhoea from any cause because marked mucosal hyperaemia may be present in the absence of specific colonic disease. Homosexual men often have non-specific cellular infiltration in the lamina propria, without pathological significance.

References

McMillan A, Lee FD. Sigmoidoscope and microscopic appearances of the rectal mucosa in homosexual men. *Gut* 1981; **22**: 1035–41

Holdstock G, Savage D, Harman M, Wright R. An investigation into the validity of the rectal classification of inflammatory bowel disease. *Q J Med* 1985; **54**: 183–90

Reynolds JR, Armitage NC, Balfour TW, Hardcastle JD. Flexible sigmoidoscopy as out-patient procedure. *Lancet* 1983; **2**: 1072

Kalra L, Price WR, Jones BJM, Hamlyn AN. Open access fibresigmoidoscopy: a comparative audit of efficacy. *Br Med J* 1988; **296**: 1095–6

RECTAL BIOPSY (RIGID INSTRUMENT)

This is a simple and safe procedure and instruments capable of obtaining a biopsy should always be available when a proctosigmoidoscopy is performed.

Method

No anaesthetic is required if a biopsy is taken from the mucosa beyond the anal margin. A specimen is obtained from any growth that is seen, or from the mucosa itself, in which case it is easiest to biopsy one of the rectal valves, the uppermost being preferred. Many different biopsy forceps are available but unfortunately most are designed for biopsy tumours and it is not always possible to obtain good samples of the mucosa. A useful instrument is a 40 cm Chevalier Jackson (basket-shaped) forceps. This is introduced via the rigid proctosigmoidoscope and the area selected for biopsy is grasped. It is simple to catch a free margin of a rectal valve. The instrument is rotated gently to free the specimen and withdrawn. The sample is removed from the forceps with a needle and gently unrolled, placed on filter paper and immersed in formol-saline. The biopsy site is inspected. Usually bleeding is slight and stops rapidly, but it may be necessary to apply compression with a cotton wool swab. It is doubtful whether 1:1000 adrenalin solution applied to the area is useful. The proctosigmoidoscope is withdrawn and the patient warned that the next stool is likely to be bloodstained. Significant bleeding and perforation are uncommon complications. A few days should elapse between the taking of a biopsy and a barium enema examination.

New rectal forceps with flexible jaws containing a fixing pin have been described at St Mark's Hospital.

Other biopsy instruments that can be used include the Truelove–Salt biopsy instrument which works on the basis of suction. The instrument is advanced through a proctosigmoidoscope, and the cutting hole which is in the head of the instrument is placed on the site for biopsy. Suction is applied via a syringe and a small knuckle of mucosa is drawn into the orifice. The knife is advanced to amputate and trap the specimen.

Interpretation

Careful attention to handling, processing and sectioning is necessary to ensure accurate interpretation. Serial sections are cut perpendicular to the submucosal surface. Only the well-orientated sections are studied. Flattening the sample gently on a glass slide (or filter paper) prior to fixation assists optimal sectioning.

Normal

The glands are seen to be tubular and closely packed and the epithelium is columnar. There are numberous goblet cells. The lamina propria contains a moderate number of lymphocytes, plasma cells, reticuloendothelial cells and the occasional eosinophil. Variations within the normal range include slight dilatation or tortuosity of the glands, cuboidal surface epithelial cells and some increase in round cells in the lamina propria. The rectal glands are bulbous and shortened in specimens obtained from near the anal region.

Ulcerative colitis

In severe cases there is marked loss of glandular structure, extensive mucosal ulceration with a heavy infiltration of cells particularly polymorphonuclear leukocytes, crypt abscesses, and a reduction in goblet cells and mucus. In moderate and mild inflammation there is oedema, dilatation of vessels, an occasional crypt abscess and superficial ulceration. There is an increase in lymphocytes, plasma cells and polymorphonuclear leukocytes. There is generally good correlation between the sigmoidoscopic and histological findings but this is not always so. The biopsy specimen is more likely to show inflammation when the proctosigmoidoscopic findings are normal than the reverse. Once the disease has developed, the mucosa remains permanently abnormal in the majority of patients whether or not symptoms are present. Biopsy samples obtained during a quiescent phase show a reduction in the number of rectal glands which tend to be bulbous, tortuous and branched. There is nothing specific about the mucosal biopsy in ulcerative colitis and all the features of the mucosal alterations in this disease may be found in colitis from other causes.

Rectal biopsies are valuable in the diagnosis of precancer in patients with ulcerative colitis. There are two main types of abnormality: the polypoid variety, and precancerous change in a flat mucosa. *Polypoid precancerous changes* are recognized by the presence of multiple polyps which are usually sessile with a villous or papillary surface configuration. The villous growth pattern is the more significant. There is obvious inflammation in the lamina propria with loss of goblet cells. The nuclei are hyperchromatic with many mitotic figures. *Precancerous change in a flat mucosa* is more common. The mucosa is thicker and has a fairly nodular surface. The epithelial tubes are irregular in shape and size with lateral budding and a villous growth pattern. There is a tendency for the epithelial tubes to proliferate into the submucosa. A moderate amount of inflammatory cell infiltration is present. The implication of these histological features in the management of chronic ulcerative colitis remains uncertain.

Granulomatous colitis (Crohn's disease of the colon)

The mucosa is either normal or shows non-specific inflammatory changes. It is helpful but unusual to find non-caseating giant-cell systems in the biopsy specimen.

Tumours

A papillary or villous *adenoma* will show a broad base with characteristic long papillary projections springing almost directly from the basement membrane. An adenomatous *polyp* shows focal glandular hyperplasia; there may be short papillary projections but there are always numerous glands below the surface epithelium and the villi do not extend to the submucosal base. The stalk is often fibromuscular in character. *Colonic cancers* are usually adenocarcinomas and less frequently colloid cancers.

Schistosomiasis

It is claimed that in light infections with *S. mansoni* some 50% or more patients will be diagnosed if rectal biopsies are taken than if only the stools are examined. Rectal biopsies are useful also in *S. haematobium* infections. The ova are easily recognized when a fresh unstained biopsy of mucosa is compressed between two glass slides and examined under the microscope.

Rectal biopsies have been used to advantage in the diagnosis of amoebic colitis, amyloidosis, histiocytosis, some of the neurolipidoses and metachromatic leukodystrophy. *Hirschsprung's disease* can be detected with the use of special stains for nerve fibres and acetycholinesterase activity.

References

Morson BC, Pang LSC. Rectal biopsy as an aid to cancer control in ulcerative colitis. *Gut* 1967; **8**: 423–34

Riddell RH, Morson BC. Value of sigmoidoscopy and biopsy in detection of carcinoma and premalignant change in ulcerative colitis. *Gut* 1979; **20**: 575–80

Leonard-Jones JE, Misiewicz JJ, Parrish JA, Ritchie JK, Swarbrick ET, Williams CB. Prospective study of out-patients with extensive colitis. *Lancet* 1974; **i**: 1065–9

Cook MC, Goligher JC. Carcinoma and epithelial dysplasia complicating ulcerative colitis. *Gastroenterology* 1975; **68**: 1127–36

Dickinson RJ, Gilmour HM, McClelland DBL. Rectal biopsy in patients presenting to an infectious disease unit with diarrhoeal disease. *Gut* 1979; **20**: 141–8

Jass JR, Love SB, Northover JMA. A new prognosis classification of rectal cancer. *Lancet* 1987; **1**: 1303–6

Nostrant TT, Kumar NB, Appleman HD. Histopathology differentiates acute self-limited colitis from ulcerative colitis. *Gastroenterology* 1987; **92**: 318–28

Barr LC, Booth J, Filipe MI, Lawson JON. Clinical evaluation of the histochemical diagnosis of Hirschsprung disease. *Gut* 1985; **26**: 393–9

Preston DM, Butt JH, Lennard-Jones JE, Morson BC. New rectal-mucosal biopsy forceps. *Lancet* 1983; **1**: 157

RADIOLOGY

Radiological examination is important in the diagnosis of colonic disease, despite advances in endoscopic techniques.

Plain abdominal radiograph

The plain radiograph of the abdomen is helpful in acute, toxic ulcerative colitis when varying degrees of colonic dilatation may be seen as well as other features of ulcerative colitis such as loss of haustrations and large pseudopolyps. The site of a colonic cancer may be suspected when there is an abrupt end to the colonic gas shadow. In ischaemic colitis there may be gas in abnormal sites, such as the bowel wall, and evidence of mucosal oedema ('thumb printing').

Barium enema (Figures 15–18)

A barium enema is usually required in the diagnosis of disease in the colon. It is important that the radiologist is given ample clinical information, particularly when ulcerative colitis or diverticulitis is suspected because the technique of preparation and examination may have to be modified. As a rule a barium enema should not be performed in acute ulcerative colitis or acute diverticulitis. The examination is not without danger, and it can exacerbate the colitis or cause a perforation of an acutely inflamed bowel. When a barium enema is performed it should routinely include air-contrast studies because these give far superior results and leave fewer uncertainties to be resolved by colonoscopy.

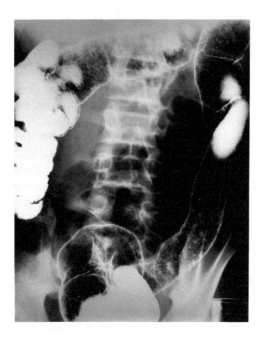

Figure 15 Barium enema showing total ulcerative colitis

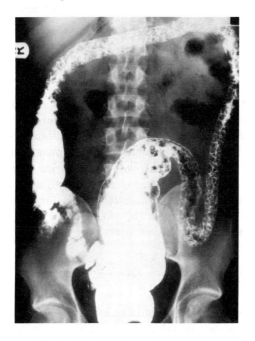

Figure 16 Barium enema showing pancolitis due to Crohn's disease-typical 'cobblestone appearance

Interpretation

Ulcerative colitis

There are fine serrations along the bowel margin, loss of haustrations, pseudopolyps and extensive undermining of the mucosa. In longstanding disease there may be loss of haustrations, marked shortening of the bowel and rigidity producing the typical 'hose-pipe' colon; on the other hand the radiographic appearances may be virtually normal. In mild colitis flattening and blunting of the haustration give a 'corrugated' appearance. It must be remembered that a normal colon may have no haustration distal to the splenic flexure. Changes in the rectum of diagnostic value include thickening and irregularity of the mucosal folds, small ulcerations, and contraction of the rectal wall. There is an increase in the retrorectal soft tissue space which is greater than 10 mm. A barium enema is of value in determining the extent of the colonic involvement in ulcerative colitis.

While there is a good correlation in general between the colonoscopic, histological and radiological findings in this disease, this is not always so. Disease defined by colonoscopy tends to be more extensive than that seen by radiology. It is advisable that the diagnosis of ulcerative colitis be made on the basis of all three investigations. Regrettably, the barium enema usually demonstrates a carcinoma superimposed upon ulcerative colitis only at a fairly advanced stage of growth.

Granulomatous (Crohn's) colitis

At an early stage there are ileal and caecal impressions due to swollen lymph nodes at the ileocaecal junction, a decrease in the caecal lumen and reversible narrowing of the colonic lumen associated with small ulcers. At a more advanced stage the involvement is seen to be segmental, there is thickening and blunting of the mucosal folds with asymmetrical involvement. Inflammatory polyps, linear and transverse ulcerations, pseudodiverticula and stricture formation may all be seen. Characteristically, the right side of the colon is more frequently involved than the left. However, Crohn's disease may closely mimic ulcerative colitis.

Neoplastic lesions

In the colon these appear as cicatrizing lesions or as proliferative 'polypoid' growths. The incidence of false-negative diagnosis in cancer of the colon (excluding the rectum) is about 10%. The site of the cancer determines to some extent whether or not it is detected. Growths in the rectum and at the

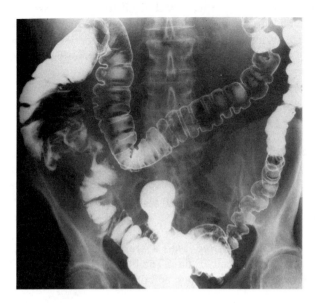

Figure 17 Double-contrast barium enema showing a large filling defect in the caecum due to carcinoma

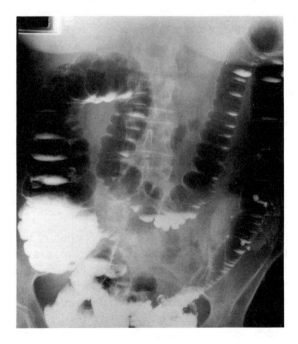

Figure 18 Double contrast barium enema showing diverticular disease in the sigmoid, descending and ascending colon

rectosigmoid junction are particularly difficult to see, and associated diverticular disease adds to the difficulties. The Malmö technique, a modification of the double contrast method in which special attention is given to direct preparation of the colon, has a very high detection rate for colonic polypoid tumours.

Other diseases

Diverticular disease. The diverticula usually fill with barium. A jagged 'sawtooth' appearance with apparently marked mucosal distortion represents failure of the colon to elongate because of muscle hypertrophy and is not evidence of inflammation. When inflammation is present there is narrowing, rigidity and intramural sinus tracts.

In the chronic stage of *ischaemic colitis* a stricture may be seen which characteristically involves the splenic flexure. The bowel may show a scalloped edge with mucosal irregularity, sacculation and tubular narrowing.

In acute *amoebiasis* shallow ulcers may be demonstrated and the appearances are those of ulcerative colitis. In the more chronic phase a contracted caecum may be seen or an amoeboma shows as a filling-defect, usually in the caecum or rectum. This condition is not usually diagnosed by radiology.

Cathartic colon. This shows an absence of normal haustral markings, a smooth bowel wall with no irregularity, no thickening of the bowel and very characteristically, pseudostrictures which are tapering, transient contractions. The changes are found initially in the right side of the colon. Proctosigmoidoscopic demonstration of melanosis coli confirms the aetiology.

ARTERIOGRAPHY

This has enjoyed a resurgence with the appreciation of the great frequency with which angiodysplasia of the right side of the colon causes rectal bleeding in the elderly. Rapid serial radiographs are taken over 30 sec, after injection of contrast medium into the superior mesenteric artery. Arterial, capillary and venous phases of filling are demonstrated. In angiodysplasia there are small clusters of arteries on the antimesenteric border of the caecum and the ascending colon, intense capillary filling, and early, intense and prolonged opacifications of the veins. It is of interest that aortic valve disease is frequently seen in patients with angiodysplasia.

Arteriography can diagnose and localize tumours of the colon, but it has largely been superseded by colonoscopy for this purpose.

References

Wellin S. Results of the Malmö technique of colon examination. *J Am Med Assoc* 1967; **199**: 369–71

Baum S, Athanasoulis CA, Waltman AC, Galdabini J, Schapiro RH, Warshaw AL, Ottinger LW. Angiodysplasia of the right colon: A cause of gastrointestinal bleeding. *Am J Roentgenol* 1977; **129**: 789–94

Fork FT. Double contrast enema and colonoscopy in polyp detection. *Gut* 1981; **22**: 971–7

COLONOSCOPY

The direct inspection of the mucosa of the whole large bowel has contributed greatly to understanding of colonic disease.

The essentials for adequate examination are a clean colon and a co-operative patient, satisfactory barium enema films, an image intensifier, and modern fibreoptic instruments.

If all these conditions are met it is possible to examine fully the left side of the colon in almost every patient, and in 70% or more of examinations the caecum is reached. The procedure is, however, difficult and time-consuming. Success depends on operator experience, and it is common for the initial examinations by an investigator to be very frustrating.

Instruments

The equipment for colonoscopy is shown in Figures 19–21. There is a range of lengths of instruments. Among the most useful are those of length 140 cm and 180 cm. These have a single biopsy and suction channel. If it is only desired to inspect the sigmoid and descending colon then 60 and 100 cm instruments may be used, as they are more easily manoeuvred. Biopsy forceps are available for the various colonoscopes. Other useful accessories include a diathermy snare and polyp-grasping forceps and a CO_2 insufflator for polypectomy.

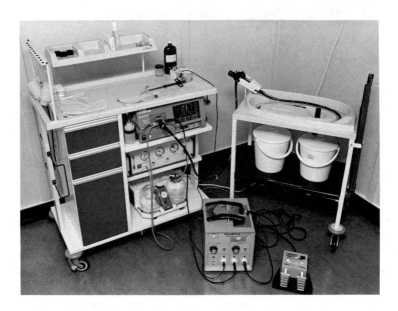

Figure 19 Colonoscopy trolley and diathermy snare equipment

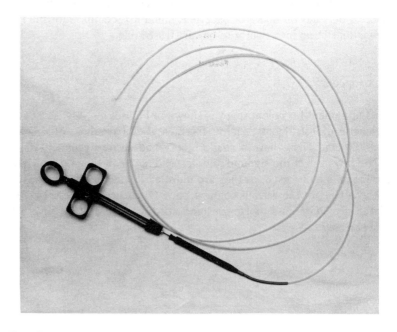

Figure 20(a) Polypectomy snare in sheath

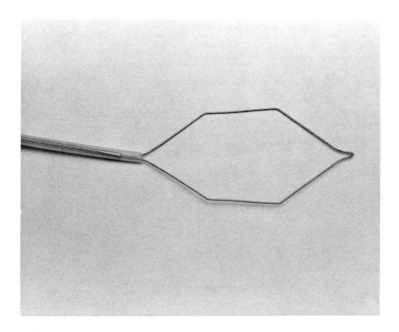

Figure 20(b) Polypectomy snare

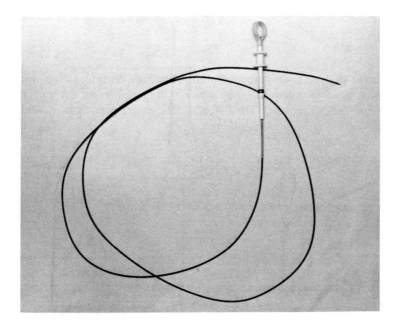

Figure 21(a) Polyp forceps in sheath

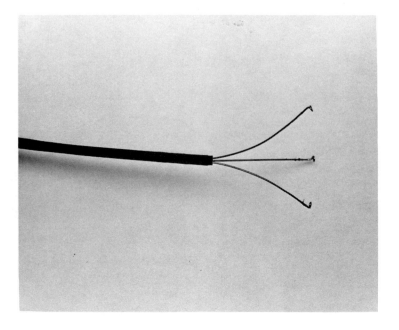

Figure 21(b) Polyp grasping tripod forceps

Preparation

The procedure is discussed with the patient and an explanation given for the importance of adequate preparation. Preparation usually begins 3 days before the examination. The following scheme is generally successful:

> *Day 1* Clear fluids only by mouth.
> Sennosides by mouth in the afternoon with a glass of water.
> *Day 2* Clear fluids only by mouth.
> *Day 3* Nil by mouth.
> Enema (1-2 litres) water in the morning at least 3 hours before the examination.

This scheme requires modification in children. It must not be used in patients with severe relapses of inflammatory bowel disease in whom colonoscopy is rarely indicated. If a patient has had appreciable bleeding, the bowel is often empty of faeces and no preparation is necessary.

Alternative preparation (Golytely)

A safe technique involves the use of sodium sulphate lavage. A solution is made up with sodium sulphate, and polyethylene glycol (80 mM) to give an electrolyte concentration in mEq/l of: Na 125; K 10; SO_4 80; Cl 35; HCO_3 20. This may be flavoured and 2.5–5.0 litres are drunk; or a nasogastric tube is passed and the patient is placed on a comfortable lavatory seat. The solution is then infused at 20–30 ml/min, and purgation is complete in 3 hours. This preparation is rapid and obviates the need for any preliminaries before the day of colonoscopy. The solution used is stated not to permit any appreciable net fluid secretion or absorption in the intestine.

Physiological saline and mannitol purges proved hazardous and they should not be used.

Procedure

The patient is positioned in the left lateral position with the knees drawn up and the buttocks on the edge of the bed.

A rectal examination is performed to ensure that there are no faeces present. Midazolam 10 mg and pethidine 50 mg i.v. are given slowly. The dose may need reduction in the elderly or respiratory invalid, and naloxone 400 mcg and flumazenil 500 mcg should be available to reverse excess sedation. The lubricated instrument is introduced into the rectum and the light switched on to visualize the mucosa. If the bowel lumen is not clearly seen, gentle air insufflation and withdrawal are helpful. The view may be partly obscured by traces of residual faeces or enema, but it is not worthwhile trying to clear the field completely. The lumen is followed as far as possible, using the directional controls, torsion and withdrawal. If the lumen cannot be brought into view, progress can nonetheless be made by 'sliding by' the mucosa, but should the mucosa blanch or fail to move past the lens the instrument should be withdrawn a little. The *sigmoid colon* is tortuous and navigation is especially difficult in the presence of diverticular disease. Loops may be formed which prevent progress even when the lumen is well in view. Torsion and withdrawal usually improves the position.

Once the *descending colon* is reached it is usually possible to straighten out the sigmoid colon by judicious withdrawal and making the sigmoid colon concertina on the instrument. The success of this manoeuvre can be checked by rolling the patient on to the back and visualizing the position of the colonoscope using the image intensifier.

In cases of difficulty in negotiating the sigmoid colon the 'alpha loop' manoeuvre may be helpful. The instrument is withdrawn to the lower sigmoid and the colonoscope twisted 180° anticlockwise before further entry. This creates a single spiral in the sigmoid and permits further passage up into the descending colon. The loop must be undone by clockwise rotation when the tip is in the descending colon.

The descending colon is straight and usually traversed with ease. The *splenic flexure* is variable in conformity; it may be passed readily but often it is a sharp angle which necessitates much manipulation and air insufflation for passage. The dusky purplish appearance of the spleen and/or liver may be seen through the upper part of the splenic flexure and is a helpful landmark. The *transverse colon* is triangular in shape and freely mobile. It is possible to stretch the bowel without making progress in which event the instrument should be cautiously withdrawn, whereupon paradoxical advance of the tip is often seen. The *hepatic flexure* can be identified by the purplish appearance of the adjacent liver, but this part of the bowel is even more variable than the splenic flexure and may be passed without being identified. The *ascending colon* is quite short and easily negotiated. If it appears that there is insufficient length of instrument to pass the whole colon, it is helpful to withdraw and suck out air. The *caecum* is recognized by the fact that it is a cul-de-sac, often with prominent folds. It contains the ileocaecal valve and appendix orifice, but neither of these is invariably seen, and it is essential to confirm by fluoroscopy that the whole colon has been passed. It is sometimes possible to enter the terminal ileum. The mucosa is inspected during withdrawal of the instrument and, in order to avoid loops rushing by the tip of the endoscope, it should be removed gradually.

Interpretation

Inflammatory bowel disease can be classified by colonoscopy according to its extent and severity. In *ulcerative coliltis* there is a uniform inflammation of the mucosa which almost always affects the rectum and spreads proximally continuously. Frank bleeding may be seen, but the separate ulcers are too small to identify. In *Crohn's disease* similar appearances can occur, but often there are discrete ulcers with relatively normal mucosa in between. Rectal spasm and discontinuous disease are common in Crohn's colitis. *Amoebiasis* appears as raised ulcers overlying small amoebic abscesses.

Diverticular disease causes problems in passing the sigmoid colon, which is tortuous and with prominent circular muscles. The mouths of the diverticula can usually be identified and sometimes may be so large as to simulate the bowel lumen.

Vascular abnormalities (angiodysplasias) in the right side of the colon are increasingly being recognized as a cause of rectal bleeding in the elderly. They are seen as small leashes of vessels and venous lakes.

Strictures and carcinomas are usually easily recognized; biopsies should always be taken.

Polyps are a very common finding. Small 2–3 mm sessile metaplastic polyps are common and of no significance. Larger and pedunculated polyps should be biopsied or removed by diathermy snare. In practice it is only polyps greater than 10 mm in diameter which are likely to be malignant.

If the diathermy snare is used it is important to lift the polyp away from the bowel wall, to insufflate with carbon dioxide before diathermy and to ensure that there is no persistent local bleeding. The separated polyp is retrieved by forceps and submitted to histology.

Indications

(1) Evaluation and biopsy of strictures and polyps suspected of malignancy.
(2) Assessment of the extent and nature of inflammatory bowel disease.
(3) Determination of the cause of rectal bleeding, either as an immediate investigation or when the barium enema has been unhelpful.
(4) Assessment of postoperative appearances, for example tumour recurrence, activity of inflammatory bowel disease prior to anastomosis.
(5) Diagnostic and therapeutic polypectomy without laparotomy.
(6) Identification of luminal lesions at open surgery.
(7) Exclusion of multiple diseases, e.g. inflammatory bowel disease and coexisting diverticular disease.
(8) Confirmation of ischaemic colitis.
(9) Inspection of the terminal ileum in suspected Crohn's disease.

Cleansing

Cleansing is performed in a manner similar to that used for upper digestive endoscopes. Thorough washing is essential and a very soft toothbrush or cotton buds are helpful in cleaning the lens. Social hygiene is the ideal, and any attempt to 'sterilize' a dirty instrument in between the examination of patients on a list will prove to be valueless.

References

Davis GR, Sant Ana CA, Morawski SG, Fordtran JS. Development of a lavage solution associated with minimal water and electrolyte absorption or secretion. *Gastroenterology* 1980; **78**: 991–5

Overholt BF. Colonoscopy. A review. *Gastroenterology* 1975; **68**: 1308–20

Shinya H, Wolff WI. Colonoscopic polypectomy: technique and safety. *Hosp Prac* 1975; **10**: 71–8

Durdey P, Weston PMT, Williams NS. Colonoscopy or barium enema as initial investigation of colonic disease. *Lancet* 1987; **2**: 549–51

MANOMETRY

Pressure recordings may be obtained from the colon and anorectal region by balloons, open-ended (fluid-filled) catheters and radiotelemetry capsules with pressure sensors. There is a wide overlap in the pressures obtained in normal and in disease states, but manometry can help in diagnosis and in monitoring progress. Results are observer-dependent, as in oesophageal manometry. *Motility* can be measured by following the progress of radio-opaque shapes, by radiotelemetry capsules and by the use of free or encapsulated ^{51}chromium.

The *normal* colonic motor activity includes segmental contractions and mass movements. The pressure waves measured by balloons and catheters reflect unco-ordinated non-propulsive segmental contractions, with an amplitude of 10–60 mm mercury. They are present for 50% of the time and are apparently random. They are increased by food, cholinergic stimuli and probably cholecystokin. They are decreased by atropine, catecholamines, prostaglandin E_2 and during sleep.

Segmental activity is reduced in *diarrhoeal states*, and increased in *constipation, diverticular disease* and the *irritable bowel syndrome*.

Measurement of anorectal pressures can be used in the diagnosis of *Hirschsprung's disease*. In normal controls, balloon distension of the rectum leads to reflex relaxation of the internal anal sphincter (smooth muscle) and contraction of the external anal sphincter (striated muscle). In Hirschsprung's disease there is no relaxation, or even actual contraction, of the internal sphincter. This does not occur in idiopathic megacolon or other diseases. The diagnosis of Hirschsprung's disease can be confirmed by the absence of the autonomic nerve plexus on rectal biopsy samples which also contain abnormally high acetylcholinesterase activity (normals up to 10.9 units/g tissue; Hirschsprung's disease 16.9–63.0 units/g tissue).

Abnormalities of anorectal pressure have also been reported in idiopathic constipation and in incontinence.

References

Holdstock DJ, Misiewicz JJ. Factors controlling colonic motility: colonic pressures and transit after meals in patients with total gastrectomy, pernicious anaemia or duodenal ulcer. *Gut* 1970; **11**: 100–10

Aaronson I, Nixon HH. A clinical evaluation of anorectal pressure studies in the diagnosis of Hirschsprung's disease. *Gut* 1972; **13**: 138–46

Dale G, Bonham JR, Lowdon P, Wagget J, Rangecroft L, Scott DJ. Diagnostic value of rectal mucosal acetylcholinesterase levels in Hirschsprung's disease. *Lancet* 1979; i: 347–9

Keighley MRB, Buchmann P, Lee JR. Assessment of anorectal function in selection of patients for ileorectal anastomosis in Crohn's colitis. *Gut* 1982; **23**: 102–7

Read NW, Haynes WG, Bartolo DCC *et al.* Use of anorectal manometry during rectal infusion of saline to investigate sphincter function in incontinent patients. *Gastroenterology* 1983; **85**: 105–13

Narducci F, Bassotti G, Gaburri M, Morelli A. 24-hour manometric recording of colonic motor activity in healthy man. *Gut* 1987; **28**: 17–25

Metcalfe AM, Phillips SF, Zinsheister AR, MacCarty RC, Beart RW, Wolff BG. Simplified assessment of segmental colonic transit. *Gastroenterology* 1987; **92**: 40–7

Akervall S, Nordgren S, Oresland T, Hulten L. Manovolumetry: a new method for investigation of anorectal function. *Gut* 1988; **29**: 614–23

Leigh RJ, Turnberg LA. Faecal incontinence: the unvoiced symptom. *Lancet* 1982; **1**: 1349–52

IMMUNOLOGY

Inflammatory bowel disease

Despite the probable disorder of immune mechanisms present in ulcerative colitis and Crohn's disease, immunological studies have not proved useful in diagnosis. Fifteen percent of patients with ulcerative colitis have antibodies to colonic epithelial cell cytoplasm, and in rather more there are IgG-class antireticulin antibodies. Patients with associated liver disease will have antismooth muscle and antimitochondrial antibodies. A high frequency of the human leukocyte antigen HLA-B27 is observed when ankylosing spondylitis occurs in association with inflammatory bowel disease. Haemagglutinating antibodies can be found, especially in children, and are not necessarily linked with autoimmune haemolytic anaemia. The acute phase reactant alpha-acid glycoprotein (orosomucoid) and haptoglobin are elevated in ulcerative colitis, and this correlates with clinical activity of the disease. By contrast prealbumin tends to fall in active ulcerative colitis.

Carcinoembryonic antigen (CEA)

This glycoprotein was first found in tumour tissue from patients with large bowel cancer, and it was later shown to be present in serum as well.

It is detected in 50–90% of patients with large bowel cancer. When an upper limit of normal of 5 mcg/l is set, only 1.1% of healthy non-smoking individuals have CEA in their serum. However, it is commonly found in apparently healthy smokers in the range 5–17 mcg/l, and also in patients with carcinomas of the lung, pancreas and gastrointestinal tract, in severe alcoholic liver disease and in anaemia. It therefore has limited value as a screening test.

CEA levels usually fall to normal in patients whose large bowel carcinoma has been completely resected and who have no metastases. A subsequent rise in titre indicates recurrent tumour, and this can be detected months before clinical recurrence. Falls in CEA levels correlate with objective response to chemotherapy in 75% of patients.

Monoclonal antibodies are under evaluation for tumour localization.

Amoebiasis

Entamoeba histolytica infection may be asymptomatic, or it may cause dysentery and liver abscesses. The stool should be examined for motile amoebae and cysts, and proctosigmoidoscopy can show typical appearances and yield diagnostic histology. However, there is often difficulty in confirming a diagnosis, and serology can be very helpful. A complement fixation test is available. It is not as helpful as indirect haemagglutination (IHA) and gel diffusion precipitation (GDP), and a combination of these two is used diagnostically. Results are shown in Table 2.

E. histolytica may be an innocent commensal, especially in the homosexual male, and zymodeme typing by electrophoresis is useful to assess pathogenicity.

Table 2 Diagnosis of amoebiasis

	Positive (%)	
	GDP	*IHA*
Amoebic liver abscess	85	95
Amoebic colitis	91	95
Other diarrhoea or liver abscesses	1	5
After effective treatment	Usually becomes negative at 6 months	Remains positive

References

Marner I-L, Friborg S, Simonsen E. Disease activity and serum proteins in ulcerative colitis. Immunochemical quantitation. *Scand J Gastroenterol* 1975; **10**: 537 – 44

Mach J-P, Jaeger P, Bertholet M-M, Ruegsegger C-H, Loosli RM, Rettavel J. Detection of recurrence of large bowel carcinoma by radioimmunoassay of circulating carcinoembryonic antigen (CEA). *Lancet* 1974; **2**: 535 – 40

Findlay IG, McArdie DS. Role of CEA in detection of asymptomatic disseminated disease in colorectal carcinoma. *Br Med J* 1983; **286**: 1242 – 4

Regent RHJ. The value of CEA in clinical practice. *Br J Hosp Med* 1987; April 335 – 8

Farrand PA, Perkins AC, Pimm MV *et al.* Radioimmunodetection of human colorectal cancers by an anti-tumour monoclonal antibody. *Lancet* 1982; **2**: 397–400

Patterson M, Healy GR, Shabot JM. Serologic testing for amoebiasis. *Gastroenterology* 1980; **78**: 136–41

Nanda R, Baveja U, Anand BS. *Entamoeba histolytica* cyst passers: clinical features and outcome in untreated subjects. *Lancet* 1984; **2**: 301–3

Goldmeer D, Sargeaunt PG, Price AB *et al.* Is *Entamoeba histolytica* in homosexual men a pathogen? *Lancet* 1986; **1**: 641–4

Weller IVA. The gay bowel. *Gut* 1985; **26**: 869–75

Stool examination

It is no longer fashionable for clinicians to make a detailed inspection of the stool. Usually more is gained from a chemical analysis of faeces, for example, for fat, haemoglobin, porphyrins and, at times, water and electrolytes. But there are occasions when to confirm that a patient's account of diarrhoea, blood, mucus or worms is correct, it is necessary to see the stools.

MACROSCOPIC APPEARANCE

Normally the stool is firm or semi-formed and is coloured varying shades of brown. It may be possible to recognize undigested food particles and their frequency reflects the nature of the diet, the amount of mastication and the degree of intestinal hurry. The shape of the stool varies greatly and is of little diagnostic significance.

Blood from anorectal diseases is seen as streaks on the surface of the stool. Blood from lesions higher up the colon will be intimately mixed with the stool as is characteristically found in inflammatory bowel disease. The passage of pure blood with no faecal material may occur with polyps, haemorrhoids, colonic cancer, diverticular disease, infarction of the colon and intussusception. Patients with bleeding peptic ulcers occasionally pass bright red, unaltered blood per rectum. The stools may be coloured red after the ingestion of beetroot, and also after the parenteral administration of brom-sulphthalein. In the latter circumstances the diagnosis is readily established by the addition of 0.1 mol/l hydrochloric acid to the stool which will alter from scarlet to a brown colour.

The stools are pale when there is intra- and extrahepatic cholestasis and in severe steatorrhoea. Tarry black melaena stools indicate the partial digestion of blood in the gastrointestinal tract. The appearance is usually characteristic, but if there is any doubt the stool is mixed with a small volume of water which will be coloured red. Chemical tests for blood should be performed. Iron-containing stools are grey-black and can usually be distinguished from melaena. Other causes of black stools include the ingestion of charcoal, bismuth compounds and large quantities of liquorice.

In cholera the stools are virtually colourless and liquid, and contain flakes of mucus, shed epithelial cells and enormous numbers of the vibrios: the 'rice water' stool. A very similar appearance is seen in staphylococcal enterocolitis which may be readily diagnosed by a Gram stain of the faecal material when numerous clumps of bacteria are seen.

PROTOZOA AND HELMINTHS

Various intestinal parasites may be seen by the naked eye in the stool including tapeworms *(Taenia solium* or *saginata)*, roundworms *(Ascaris lumbricoides)*, and threadworms *(Enterobius vermicularis)*.

A microscopic examination of a stool suspension is required to diagnose pathogenic protozoa and helminthic ova. Stool can be obtained from a bedpan or other container; alternatively it is possible to use the material off the glove after performing a rectal examination. A wooden applicator is used to place a pea-sized portion of stool on a microscope dish previously moistened with two or three drops of isotonic saline. A coverslip is applied carefully to ensure that no air bubbles are trapped. The slide is scanned under low power, and particularly at the edges. *Entamoeba histolytica* and *Entamoeba coli* can exist in vegetative and multinucleate cystic forms; the biflagellate *Giardia intestinalis* may be identified, although it is more readily found in the duodenal aspirate; and *Enterobius vermicularis* can be demonstrated. Ova which may be seen include *Ascaris lumbricoides, Ankylostoma duodenale, Necator americanus, Taenia saginata, Taenia solium, Enterobius vermicularis,* and *Strongyloides stercoralis*.

It may be necessary to undertake repeated examinations of the stool. Stools should always be collected and examined before a barium examination. Commercial stool collection kits are available which contain preservatives for parasites and cysts.

A number of crystals are normally seen in the stool including triple phosphate crystals, calcium phosphate crystals, calcium oxalate crystals and less frequently crystals of calcium carbonate and calcium sulphate. They are not of diagnostic significance.

Enterobiasis (seatworm, pinworm or thread worm, *E. vermicularis*)

This condition is not usually diagnosed from an examination of the stools because the adult female parasite is seldom longer than 10 mm and the stools contain ova in only 10% of infected patients. The usual method of diagnosis is to obtain ova from the perianal skin using the transparent adhesive tape test. This test is performed preferably in the early morning and can be undertaken by parents on their children. A quarter of an inch of clear, transparent adhesive tape is pressed on one end of a microscopic slide, The tape is folded backwards with the sticky surface facing outward. The slide is directed gently into the anal verge so that the sticky surface of the tape touches the anus and

125

immediate perianal area. The slide is then removed and the tape flipped over so that the adhesive surface attaches to the slide. The tape is smoothed over carefully using tissue paper in order to remove air bubbles and wrinkles. The slide is examined under the microscope.

Amoebiasis

The search for amoebae must be made before the patient undergoes a course of antimicrobial treatment, especially metronidalole. Similarly a mineral-oil enema or a barium enema renders the stool unsuitable for the diagnosis of amoebiasis. On the other hand a dose of penicillin has been used to 'chase' the amoebae into the stool thereby increasing the chance of finding the trophozoites in the faeces.

Only fresh, warm stool is examined. Material obtained at the time of sigmoidoscopy may also be used. A 'button' of faeces is emulsified on a slide in a drop of warm normal saline. The slide may be kept warm by heating on the microscope lamp. The preparation is examined under the low power magnification. The amoebae and their multinucleate cysts are seen as refractile objects which are examined in greater detail under the high power magnification. Trophozoites of *E. histolytica* are most likely to be found in mucus and cysts are found in the more faecal parts of the stool.

Hanging drop preparation

If the faecal suspension is applied carefully to the lower surface of a warmed slide amoebic motility may be more readily observed. The examination is made by focusing up and down.

E. histolytica trophozoites show slow 'purposeful' movements and contain ingested erythrocytes. Once the specimen is cold the vegetative forms are no longer motile, and it becomes very difficult to distinguish trophozoites from macrophages which may be haematophagous but are non-motile. The vegetative forms of *Entamoeba coli* demonstrate many pseudopodia but are non-motile and non-haematophagous.

Cyst forms of *E. histolytica* are greater than 10 mcm in diameter, have a finely granular cytoplasm and have one to four nuclei. Cysts of the non-pathogenic *E. hartmanni* appear as very similar to *E. histolytica* but are usually less than 10 mcm in diameter. *Entamoeba coli* cysts have a diameter greater than 12 mcm, a coarsely granular cytoplasm and one to eight nuclei.

While it may be easy to identify a population of amoebae it may be very difficult to identify isolated parasites, and this applies particularly to the smaller trophozoites such as the 'minuta' forms of *E. histolytica*. Staining for 30 min is necessary for this, fixation in Schaudinn's fixative is recommended

126

followed by staining with the Gomori trichrome stain.

Both amoebiasis and giardiasis are more frequent in male homosexuals; 40% are infected with either or both. In HIV disease cryptosporidial diarrhoea is common.

References

Quinn TC, Stamm WE, Goddell SE et al. The polymicrobial origin of intestinal infections in homosexual men. N Engl J Med 1983; **309**: 576–82
Green EL, Miles MA, Warhurst DC. Immunodiagnostic detection of giardia antigen in faeces by a rapid visual ELISA. Lancet 1985; **2**: 691–3

BACTERIA

A sample of freshly passed stool is taken with a disposable wooden spatula and placed in a screwtop container. The stool must be free of urine. Disposable containers with plastic spatulas attached to the lid are also convenient sampling devices. The stool should be delivered to the laboratory on the day it is passed. If amoebic dysentery is suspected a warm sample of stool should be examined immediately after the specimen has been obtained.

Alternative procedures are to take stool from the glove or proctosigmoidoscope after internal examination. Rectal swabs may be useful, but it is important that they are taken from the rectum and not the perineum. This requires passage of at least an anoscope.

Samples should be cultured in a solid selective and a liquid enrichment medium, with both aerobic and anaerobic culture. A single negative culture does not exclude infection, and normally two stool samples should be sent. However, any positive results are usually obtained with the first sample. Some individuals are asymptomatic carriers of organisms.

Bacteria which are traditionally important in diarrhoeal illnesses are *Salmonella, Shigella* and *Staphylococcus*. More recently some strains of *Escherichia coli* have been shown to be pathogenic, but their detection requires serological testing not readily available.

Patients with *Salmonella* or *Shigella* in the stool usually have diarrhoea persisting over 24 hours, fever, blood in the stool, abdominal pain and nausea. In the absence of all of these features stool culture is frequently negative, and random stool cultures in patients presenting with diarrhoea are infrequently rewarding.

Campylobacter and *Clostridium difficile* are now recognized as causes of enterocolitis. *C. difficile* infection is particularly important as it may follow antibacterial therapy. It is a fastidious anaerobe which produces a cytopathic enterotoxin that can be identified in stool. Infection is one of the few diarrhoeas needing specific antibacterial therapy.

Despite the practical problems involved in processing stool, *tuberculosis* (TB, tubercle infection) can sometimes be diagnosed by microscopy or culture, but the presence of TB bacilli in stool does not always imply enteric infection. There are only two clinical situations in which a Gram stain of the faeces is of value: staphylococcal enterocolitis and cholera.

References

Blaser MJ, Berkowitz ID, La Force FM, Cravens J, Reller LB, Wang W-II. *Camplobacter enteritis*: clinical and epidemiological features. *Ann Intern Med* 1979; **91**: 179 – 85

Larson HE, Parry JV, Price PR, Dolby J, Tyrrell DAJ. Undescribed toxin in pseudomembranous colitis. *Br Med J* 1977; **1**: 1246 – 8

Bartlett JG. Antibiotic-associated colitis. *Clin Gastroenterol* 1979; **8**: 783 – 801

Sack RB. Human diarrhoeal disease caused by enterotoxigenic *E. coli. Annu Rev Microbiol* 1975; **29**: 333 – 53

Merson MH, Rowe B, Black RE, Huq I, Gross RJ, Eusof A. Use of antisera for identification of enterotoxigenic *E. coli. Lancet* 1980; **2**: 222 – 4

Greenfield C, Ramirez JR, Pounder RE *et al. Clostridium difficile* and inflammatory bowel disease. *Gut* 1983; **24**: 713 – 7

VIRUSES

Many apparently infective diarrhoeas cannot be ascribed to a specific organism. They are commonly attributed to viral infection, though this is rarely proved. Examination of *paired sera* taken during the first acute illness and then 2 – 4 weeks later may show diagnostic elevation of titres of antibodies to viruses such as the *Coxsackie group*.

Rotavirus infection is common in children and clumped virions may be found after low-speed centrifugation of stool suspensions. Virus particles are concentrated with a selectively absorbent hydrophilic gel prior to diagnostic electron microscopy.

Electron microscopy may also reveal the presence of other viruses, in particular the 29 nm RNA particles of *Hepatitis type A*.

References

Whitby H, Rodgers FG. Detection of virus particles by electron microscopy with polyacrylamide hydrogel. *J Clin Pathol* 1980; **33**: 484 – 7

Barnett W. Viral gastroenteritis. *Med Clin N Am* 1983; **67**: 1031 – 58

Cline BL. Current drug regimes for treatment of intestinal helminth infections. *Med Clin N Am* 1982; **66**: 721 – 42

Pancreas

The investigation for pancreatic disease remains problematical and unsatisfactory despite the introduction of a host of techniques. The use of endoscopic retrograde cholangiopancreatography (ERCP), ultrasonography or computerized tomography to define the anatomy of the gland, coupled with one of the tests of exocrine secretion is probably the most satisfactory method of assessment. Estimation of steatorrhoea, glucose tolerance and serum amylase can provide valuable additional information. These tests are required to decide whether pancreatic disease is present, and if so to determine its nature. The differentiation of chronic pancreatitis from pancreatic cancer is an important though often unresolved question. The laboratory diagnosis of pancreatic disease can be quite simple in the presence of jaundice, glycosuria or steatorrhoea; it is when the only symptom is abdominal pain that the diagnosis frequently proves extremely difficult.

References

Arvanitakis C, Cooke AR. Diagnostic tests of exocrine pancreatic function and disease. *Gastroenterology* 1978; **74**: 932–48
Lankisch PG. Exocrine pancreatic function tests. *Gut* 1988; **23**: 777–98

ULTRASONOGRAPHY

The introduction of this technique has greatly simplified the investigation of the pancreas. Procedures are operator dependent, but the test is non-invasive and in experienced hands the results are accurate.

Portable real-time apparatus is available for use at the bedside. High-resolution real-time ultrasonography is currently the optimal method.

Fasting patients are examined in three main positions: prone, lateral decubitus, and supine. This permits full visualization of the whole pancreas. Sometimes effervescent preparations are necessary to fill the stomach with gas and enhance contrast. A complete record with serial transverse and sagittal sections takes about 1 hour to complete. The simultaneous use of ultrasonic scanning permits fine-needle aspiration of pancreatic lesions for cytological examination.

Interpretation

Normal pancreas reflects few echoes, and interference from other structures, gaseous distension and obesity, can be a problem. The gland may be difficult to locate because of its small size and variable position. It can be identified in about 80% of individuals.

Acute pancreatitis. The thickness of the pancreas increases to about twice normal and the parenchymal echoes lessen or disappear. More importantly the development of abscesses and pseudocysts can be readily detected in acute pancreatitis, and their progress followed by serial scans. The pancreatic scan is abnormal in 58% of patients with acute pancreatitis, and in as many as 92% whose symptoms and signs suggest a *pseudocyst*, when ultrasonography is the best method for diagnosis.

Chronic pancreatitis. The gland often but not always enlarges, and irregular areas of high and low echoes are characteristic. Calcification gives scattered foci of dense echoes, and this can be detected in about one-third of patients. Positive scans are more often found during clinical relapse. Pancreatic duct abnormalities associated with chronic pancreatitis may be detectable; an increase in calibre up to 2 cm can be found. Although a diagnostic accuracy of 65–94% can be achieved in chronic pancreatitis the method is not entirely foolproof because carcinoma of the pancreas may give similar changes.

Pancreatic carcinoma. This can be recognized in about 85% of cases as a well-defined tumour with few internal echoes. Growths above 12 mm should be detected, but there is often associated enlargement of the gland or chronic pancreatitis which makes interpretation more difficult. It is easier to diagnose tumours in the body and tail than in the head of the pancreas.

Hepatic metastases can be detected in most cases where they are present.

Obstructive jaundice. Ultrasonography should detect dilated extrahepatic ducts in 95% of cases, and when the cause lies in the pancreas its nature can be defined in the vast majority of patients.

Indications

(1)   First investigation for chronic disease where the pancreas is under suspicion.
(2)   First investigation for cholestatic jaundice (in association with hepatobiliary scans).
(3)   Diagnosis of pancreatic pseudocysts and abscesses.

(4)   Diagnosing and monitoring acute pancreatitis.

(5)   Guiding percutaneous pancreatic biopsy.

Computed tomography is definitely superior to ultrasound for non-invasive investigation of morphology.

References

Russell JGB, Vallon AG, Braganza JM, Howatt HT. Ultrasonic scanning in pancreatic disease. *Gut* 1978; **19**: 1027–33

Duncan JG, Imrie CW, Blumgart LH. Ultrasound in the management of acute pancreatitis. *Br J Radiol* 1976; **49**: 858–62

Mackie CR, Cooper MJ, Lewis MH, Moossa AR. Non-operative differentiation between pancreatic cancer and chronic pancreatitis. *Ann Surg* 1979; **189**: 480–7

Lees WR, Vallon AG, Denyer ME, Vahl SP, Cotton PB. Prospective study of ultrasonography in chronic pancreatic disease. *Br Med J* 1979; **i**: 162–4

Foster PN, Mitchell CJ, Robertson DRC *et al.* Prospective comparison of three non-invasive tests for pancreatic disease. *Br Med J* 1984; **289**: 13–6

ENDOSCOPIC RETROGRADE CHOLANGIOPANCREATOGRAPHY (ERCP)

The method is described in Chapter 2. Depending upon the circumstances an attempt may be made to outline only the pancreatic duct, or the biliary system as well.

Interpretation

It has been shown that clinical information improves the diagnostic accuracy of pancreatogram reporting, and should always be fully supplied.

Normal

The pancreas has a duct which passes obliquely cranially from the ampulla and then is roughly transverse. The diameter decreases smoothly and maximal figures are 6.5 mm in the head to 3 mm in the tail. The side ducts are variably filled. There is a wide variation in ductal anatomy. In addition the examination is complicated by, and may be unsatisfactory in, the annular or malfused pancreas. In elderly patients the duct system may widen up to 10 mm, and ductular ectasia and narrowing can occur without definite pathological significance.

Chronic pancreatitis

The main duct becomes dilated and tortuous. It may show strictures or contain filling defects. The earliest changes occur in the duct branches, which show variation in calibre and frank dilation, but these are difficult to detect. In advanced and calculous pancreatitis there may be complete obstruction to the proximal flow of contrast. Pancreatic fistulas can sometimes be seen. ERCP is not recommended in acute pancreatitis, although it will usually demonstrate a *pseudocyst* when it occurs.

Carcinoma

Abnormalities of the duct system such as obstruction or stenosis occur in 65–80% of patients and the diagnostic rate is highest in the group amenable to surgical removal. The collection of pure pancreatic juice for cytology at the time of ERCP improves the diagnostic rate to 92%.

Indications

(1) Evaluation of chronic and acute relapsing pancreatitis, especially detection of pancreatic ductal abnormalities or biliary calculi requiring surgical treatment.
(2) Differential diagnosis of chronic pancreatitis and carcinoma.
(3) Collection of pure pancreatic juice.

References

Reuben A, Johnson AL, Cotton PB. Is the pancreatogram reliable? A study of observer variation and error. *Br J Radiol* 1978; **51**: 956–62
Mackie CR, Dhorajiwala J, Blackstone MO, Bowie J, Moossa AR. Value of new diagnostic aids in relation to the disease process in pancreatic cancer. *Lancet* 1979; **ii**: 385–9
Hatfield ARW, Smithies A, Wilkins R, Levi AJ. Assessment of ERCP and pure pancreatic juice cytology in patients with pancreatic disease. *Gut* 1976; **17**: 14–21
Axon ATR, Classen M, Cotton PB, Cremer M, Freeny PC, Lees WR. Pancreatography in chronic pancreatitis. *Gut* 1984; **2**: 1107–12

COMPUTED TOMOGRAPHY (CT)

This technique allows a clear transverse sectional picture of the body by transmitting a series of X-rays at different angles. Equipment is expensive and not universally available. The beam is received by scintillation or ionization detectors instead of film, and the result displayed as an undistorted two-dimensional picture. Although no preparation is essential a low-residue diet may help to eliminate gas, and propantheline intramuscularly or glucagon intravenously reduce bowel motility artefacts. Dilute oral barium or iodine contrast media and i.v. iodine contrast media may be helpful to delineate adjacent bowel and blood vessels respectively. Obesity may actually improve results by provision of greater tissue contrast.

CT scanning can diagnose some pancreatic lesions missed by ultrasonography. The main indication is probably to investigate the patient where other procedures have failed, unless the procedure is readily available.

References

Fawcitt RA, Forbes W StC, Isherwood I, Braganza JM, Howat HT. Computed tomography in pancreatic disease. *Br J Radiol* 1978; **51**: 1–4

Wiggans G, Schein PS, MacDonald JS, Schellinger D, Harbert D. Computerised axial tomography for diagnosis of pancreatic cancer. *Lancet* 1976; **ii**: 233–5

ANGIOGRAPHY

Superselective angiography or phlebography can be useful ancillary investigations.

Interpretation

Acute pancreatitis. Arteries are displaced with moderate dilation and irregularity of the major vessels. There is increased vascularity, but with no alteration in capillary or venous circulation. If a pseudocyst develops the vessels become sparse and are stretched.

Chronic pancreatitis. Deformity and stenosis of the surrounding vessels with tortuosity and beading of the intrapancreatic vessels is characteristic.

Tumours. Irregular, narrowed and infiltrated vessels are seen. Carcinomas are often poorly vascularized. Angiography can be used to size tumours over 1–2 cm in diameter, and assess operability. Endocrine tumours such as insulomas are often hypervascular with a fine anastomotic pattern. They can be detected if over 1 cm in diameter, but unfortunately the tumours are usually rather small.

References

Herlinger H, Finaly DBL. Evaluation and follow-up of pancreatic arteriograms. A new role for angiography in the diagnosis of carcinoma of the pancreas. *Clin Radiol* 1978; **29**: 277–84
Deutsch V, Adar R, Jacob ET, Bank H, Moles M. Angiographic diagnosis and differential diagnosis of islet-cell tumours. *Am J Roentgenol* 1973; **119**: 121–32

OTHER RADIOLOGY

Chest X-ray

This is helpful in the diagnosis of fibrocystic disease of the pancreas when there is evidence of chronic chest infection. In acute pancreatitis basal atelectasis or a pleural effusion (often left sided) may be present.

Straight abdominal radiograph

The plain radiograph of the abdomen is helpful in acute pancreatitis. An isolated distended loop of jejunum in the upper abdomen, the 'sentinel loop', may be demonstrated or there may be absence of gas in the transverse colon, the 'colon cut-off' sign. The pancreas may be seen to be calcified and stones may be present in the duct. There may be diffuse abdominal calcification following the fat necrosis that occurs in acute pancreatic inflammation.

Barium meal

Helpful signs of pancreatic disease are pressure deformities and displacement of the stomach and duodenum. Expanding pancreatic lesions enlarge the retrogastric space and deform the posterior wall of the stomach. The indentation is smooth in the case of pseudocysts of the pancreas. In cancer the enlargement is usually slight and any infiltration of the stomach results in a rigid appearance. Changes in the gastric antrum are also seen. The duodenum may be enlarged and there may be depression of the ligament of Treitz. Pressure on the medial wall of the duodenum will give the inverted-3 sign of Frostberg which is an indication of a pancreatic mass and does not differentiate cancer from inflammation. Pressure on the lateral aspect of the duodenum with rigidity and compression may occur in pancreatic cancer.

Barium studies are seldom used to diagnose pancreatic disease.

PERITONEOSCOPY (laparoscopy)

This procedure is described in Chapter 14.

An infragastric method has been devised for diagnosis and staging pancreatic cancer. Direct visualization permits biopsy or aspiration for cytology and avoids the hazards of laparotomy.

Reference

Cuschieri A, Hall AW, Clark J. Value of laparoscopy in the diagnosis and management of pancreatic carcinoma. *Gut* 1978; **19**: 672–7

CYTOLOGY

Material for cytology may be obtained by several methods:

(1) aspiration of the pancreas by direct puncture at laparotomy or laparoscopy using a standard 21-gauge needle;

(2) a guided percutaneous puncture with a Chiba needle;

(3) collection of pancreatic juice during ERCP or duodenal intubation for the testing of pancreatic function.

At least four smears are made onto slides, which are fixed at once in 95% alcohol and stained by the Papanicolaou method. Positive results are obtained in at least 75% of pancreatic cancer patients while false-positive results are rare.

References

Shorey BA. Aspiration biopsy of carcinoma of the pancreas. *Gut* 1975; **16**: 645–7

Smith EH, Bartrum RJ, Chang YC, D'Orsi CJ, Lokich J, Abbruzzese A, Dantano J. Percutaneous aspiration biopsy of the pancreas under ultrasonic guidance. *N Engl J Med* 1975; **292**: 825–8

Osne M, Serck-Hanssen A, Kristensen O, Swensen T, Aune S, Myren J. Endoscopic retrograde brush cytology in patients with primary secondary malignancies of the pancreas. *Gut* 1979; **20**: 279–84

Hovdenak N, Lees WR, Pereira J, Beilby JOW, Cotton PB. Ultrasound-guided percutaneous fine-needle aspiration cytology of the pancreas. *Br Med J* 1982; **285**: 1183–4

Youngs GR, Agnew JE, Levin GE, Bouchier IAD. A comparative study of 4 tests of pancreatic function in the diagnosis of pancreatic disease. *Q J Med* 1973; **42**: 597–618

HORMONAL TESTS OF PANCREATIC EXOCRINE FUNCTION

The pancreatic exocrine secretions after pancreatic stimulation can be assessed directly by duodenal drainage. Secretin stimulates the output of fluid and bicarbonate by the gland and cholecystokinin-pancreozymin (CCK-PZ) stimulates the output of enzymes. A variety of function tests has evolved using one or both hormones in different doses. The normal values of a particular laboratory depend upon the procedure used and the methods for determining the enzymes in the duodenal juice. Any one of a number of variations on the basic test is satisfactory provided the laboratory consistently uses the same method, and establishes the range of normality. Completeness of collection of duodenal juice is important. This may cause problems after gastric surgery, where only a normal result is absolutely conclusive.

The many different methods which are used to stimulate pancreatic exocrine function make the comparison of pancreatic function tests difficult. It is debatable whether pancreozymin increases the diagnostic accuracy of secretin tests, and its use is associated with a significant number of reactions. On the other hand enzyme analysis is definitely meaningful after pancreozymin and many investigators find alterations in the enzyme output of the gland to be a sensitive test of pancreatic inflammatory disease.

Multiple enzyme determinations are necessary for routine clinical use. Trypsin is usually measured nowadays but either amylase or lipase are also satisfactory. Although time consuming and relatively unpleasant for the patient, a test of pancreatic exocrine secretion is probably the most sensitive index currently available for pancreatic function.

Secretin test

Method

The patient fasts overnight. A double-lumen gastroduodenal tube is passed and positioned fluoroscopically so that the tip lies in the third part of the duodenum. Alternatively, two separate nasogastric tubes can be passed, one being positioned with the tip at the third part of the duodenum and the other sited in the gastric antrum. The patient lies tilted to the left side with the head and shoulders supported by a pillow. Continuous suction is applied to both tubes at a sub-atmospheric pressure of 5 – 10 mmHg, and this is interrupted by frequent manual aspirations to ensure patency of the tubes. The patient is not required to expectorate. The gastric aspirate is discarded. The aim is to collect duodenal samples uncontaminated by gastric secretions.

A basal collection of duodenal material is made for 10 – 30 min during which time the pH must be greater than 7.5 units. This is followed by the intravenous injection over 2 min of 1.0 unit secretin/kg body weight in

10–20 ml of normal saline. Following the secretin stimulus the duodenum is aspirated continually for 60 min. The colour and pH of the gastric and duodenal aspirates are checked frequently to ensure an uncontaminated collection. The duodenal aspirate is collected into iced containers. The volume of the duodenal aspirate is recorded.

An aliquot of the pooled collection provides a satisfactory measure of pancreatic function for clinical purposes. A variation of the method is to collect and assay timed samples of the duodenal aspirates. The sample for estimation is well mixed with an equal volume of glycerol to increase enzyme stability and analysed for bicarbonate and enzyme concentration. Amylase is often measured, but a variety of other pancreatic enzymes have been studied and in general give comparable results to amylase. However, amylase is an unreliable measure of pancreatic function in infants, where trypsin provides a better index. Biliary pigment output may be recorded as + to + + + + but is of little clinical value. A search can be made for malignant cells using the cytological methods described.

Interpretation

Normal. In adults the average volumes is 3.2 ml/kg body weight with a lower limit of 2.0 ml/kg. The average bicarbonate concentration is 108 mmol/l with a lower limit of 90 mmol/l. The average amylase concentration is 14.2 units/kg body weight with a lower limit of 6.0 units/kg body weight, but results vary depending upon the method used for amylase estimation. Amylase values for infants are slightly lower than the adult range. In adults neither age nor sex influences the output of bicarbonate.

Acute pancreatitis. The secretin test is potentially hazardous and thus of little practical value.

Chronic pancreatitis. There is a reduction in the output of bicarbonate, and values as low as 30 mEq/l are recorded. The volume is usually normal but may also be reduced.

Cancer of the pancreas. In cancer involving the head and body of the gland there is a reduction in the volume of pancreatic secretion with normal bicarbonate concentration. In diffuse involvement of the gland by malignant growth there is often a reduction in total bicarbonate output. In cancer of the tail, function is usually normal.

Haemochromatosis. It is claimed that in haemochromatosis there is a high volume flow (10–20 ml/kg body weight) with a low bicarbonate.

Diabetes mellitus. Although there is some controversy the evidence suggests that in idiopathic diabetes mellitus exocrine pancreatic function may be reduced. Some studies on patients with idiopathic diabetes have revealed a number with associated chronic pancreatitis and pancreatic cancer.

Other diseases. Disturbed pancreatic function has been recorded in patients with coeliac disease, ulcerative colitis and amyotrophic lateral sclerosis. A high volume of pancreatic flow has been recorded in 50–70% of cirrhotic patients and about 40% have reduced concentrations of bicarbonate and enzymes. Alcoholic liver disease may, of course, be associated with alcoholic pancreatitis. Heavy cigarette smoking (20+ per day) will reduce pancreatic secretion.

Neither the use of CCK-PZ together with secretin, nor the further estimation of enzyme output have clearly been shown to improve the diagnostic accuracy of the secretin test.

Augmented secretin test

Method

An intravenous infusion of 2 units secretin/kg body weight is given at a rate of 1 unit/kg/min. The duodenum is aspirated for 1 hour and the volume and bicarbonate output are measured.

Interpretation

Normal subjects have a mean volume of 2.7 ml/kg body weight with a lower limit of 1.8 ml/kg body weight. The normal mean bicarbonate concentration is 78 mEq/l with a lower limit of 54 mEq/l.

In chronic pancreatitis the mean volume is 1.7 ml/kg body weight and the mean bicarbonate concentration is 25 mEq/l.

In cancer of the pancreas the mean volume output is 1.1 ml/kg body weight and the mean bicarbonate output is 36 mEq/l. This test is claimed to be the most reliable not only in distinguishing normals from patients with pancreatic disease but also in the differentiation of chronic pancreatitis from cancer, but more experience with the technique is required. The accuracy of the test is increased by relating the volume output to the body weight.

Continuous infusion of secretin

The maximum response of the pancreas to an intravenous infusion of secretin is reached at rates of 4–6 units/min. The continuous infusion of secretin in this dose for 2 hours has been suggested as a test of pancreatic exocrine function.

Test meals: the Lundh test

Attempts have been made to measure the secretion of pancreatic enzymes in response to various test meals. The test described by Lundh is the most widely used.

Method

After an overnight fast the patient swallows a tube which is screened into position so that the tip lies between the ampulla of Vater and the duodenojejunal flexure (Figure 22). Duodenal juice is drained by siphonage into a container which is kept on ice. The drainage is maintained by intermittent gentle suction.

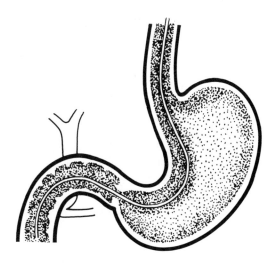

Figure 22 Position of tube for Lundh test

Once the tube is in the required position a resting sample of duodenal juice is obtained. This is followed by the administration of the test meal which comprises 18 g corn or soya bean oil, 15 g Casilan, 40 g glucose and a flavouring agent. The meal is made up to 300 ml with warm water. After ingestion of the meal the duodenum is drained over 2 hours, the samples being pooled into four collections, each of 30 min. They should be collected in containers immersed in ice and may be kept for delayed analysis by addition of an equal volume of glycerol and stored in a freezer. The pH, volume and trypsin content of the samples are measured. The four samples can be analysed separately but are more conveniently pooled and the tryptic activity expressed as the mean tryptic activity of the aspirate.

Tryptic activity is measured by a variety of methods. There is a simple method in which a measurement is made of the rate at which H^+ ions are liberated by the hydrolysis of a specific substrate N-benzoyl-L-arginine ethylester hydrochloride. This is achieved by measuring the time taken to neutralize a known amount of alkali. The results are expressed in international units (mcEq H^+/min/ml). A simple kit is available which is based on this method (Boehringer-Mannheim).

Radioimmunoassay kits have also been employed for analyses of both duodenal and serum trypsin.

Interpretation

Normal. The mean 2-hour tryptic activity is 15.4 iu with a range of 11–20 iu. In *pancreatic inflammatory disease associated with steatorrhoea* the mean tryptic activity is usually less than 2 iu. In those patients in whom the *pancreatic inflammatory disease* presents mainly as *abdominal pain* the values of tryptic activity are usually below the normal range. Low values are found in *pancreatic cancer* but equally low values may occur in *biliary obstruction* from other causes. The values are reduced for non-pancreatic causes of steatorrhoea, but they are not as low as in pancreatogenous steatorrhoea. Normal values are found in liver disease.

Using a more complex method for estimating tryptic activity, Lundh found the normal range to be 161–612 mcg trypsin/ml with a mean of 310 mcg trypsin/ml. Markedly depressed values were found in chronic pancreatitis and cancer of the pancreas.

Indications

This test is recommended because it is simple to perform and entails little discomfort for the patient. It gives reproducible results and has proved to be a reliable method in the diagnosis of chronic pancreatitis, particularly when steatorrhoea is present. It is also helpful in the diagnosis of ampullary cancer with or without jaundice. It is of little value in the retrospective diagnosis of

acute pancreatitis. However, it may be less reliable than the augmented secretin test in discriminating between the normal and abnormal pancreas.

Modifications

(1)   Zieve *et al.* introduced a meal containing 14 g corn oil, 15 g dextrose, 12 g skimmed milk powder, 218 ml skimmed milk and 8 g chocolate syrup. The volume of the meal is about 250 ml. It is introduced down the polyvinyl tube into the duodenum and aspiration of the duodenal contents is undertaken for 2 hours.

(2)   Pure pancreatic juice may also be collected by cannulation of the pancreatic duct and intravenous injection of 1 unit/kg secretin. Unfortunately the analysis of the fluid collected via ERCP is no more accurate or informative than the analysis of the duodenal aspirate.

The lactoferrin levels in patients with chronic pancreatitis (all over 900 mg/ml) are much higher than normal controls or patients with pancreatic cancer (all less than 400 mg/ml). In addition, trypsin concentrations are uniformly low in pancreatic cancer (up to 12 mcg/ml) though variable in chronic pancreatitis. The combination of tests is a very reliable method of separating cancer from chronic pancreatitis.

(3)   A modification of this method is the ratio of lactoferrin: total protein in pancreatic juice. In chronic pancreatitis this ratio $>0.5\%$, whereas in controls including normals, acute pancreatitis and carcinoma of the pancreas the ratio is $<0.03\%$.

References

Lundh G. Pancreatic exocrine function in neoplastic and inflammatory disease: a simple and reliable new test. *Gastroenterology* 1962; **47**: 275 – 80

Moeller DD, Dunn GD, Klotz AP. Comparison of the pancreozymin-secretin test and the Lundh test meal. *Am J Dig Dis* 1972; **17**: 799

Barns RJ, Elmslie RG. Comparison of methods for the estimation of trypsin in duodenal fluid. *Clin Chim Acta* 1975; **58**: 165 – 71

Mottaleb A, Kapp F, Noguera ECA, Kellock TD, Wiggins HS, Waller SL. The Lundh test in the diagnosis of pancreatic disease: a review of 5 years experience. *Gut* 1973; **14**: 835 – 41

Lake-Bakaar G, McKavanagh S, Rubio CE, Epstein D, Summerfield JO. Measurement of trypsin in duodenal juice by radio-immunoassay. *Gut* 1980; **21**: 402 – 7

Fedail SS, Harvey RF, Salmon PR, Brown P, Read AE. Trypsin and lactoferrin levels in pure pancreatic juice in patients with pancreatic disease. *Gut* 1979; **20**: 983 – 6

Multigner L, Figarella C, Samel J, Sarles J. Lactoferrin and albumin in human pancreatic juice. *Dig Dis Sci* 1980; **125**: 173 – 8

Wong LTK, Turtle S, Davidson AGF. Secretin pancreozymin stimulation test and confirmation of the diagnosis of cystic fibrosis. *Gut* 1982; **23**: 744 – 50

Tubeless oral pancreatic function tests

The goal of satisfactory tests of pancreatic secretion without the requirement for the need for intubation or handling stools has been reached. Methods are based on the pancreatic enzyme activity on bentiromide, fluorescein dilaurate and triolein. None of these tests diagnose or exclude pancreatic carcinoma.

Bentiromide ^{14}C-PABA test (Figure 23)

This is a six-hour procedure. The fasted patient voids urine and is then given by mouth 1 g benzoyl-tyrosyl-p-aminobenzoic acid (bentiromide) and 5 microcuries ^{14}C-p-aminobenzoic acid (PABA) with a test meal such as 'Casilan' 20 g.

Urine is collected for 6 hours and then excretion of PABA is measured chemically. The normal individual will excrete 50% or more of the administered dose. To check the effectiveness of intestinal absorption the excretion of ^{14}C-PABA is counted, and a normal ratio of excretion of chemical PABA to ^{14}C-PABA is greater than 0.7, wheareas in chronic pancreatitis it is less than 0.6.

Various drugs can interfere with chemical analysis, the test requires a urine collection, and radioactive material is given: this has stimulated various alternatives. The serum level of PABA 90–180 min after a dose of bentiromide 1 g should be greater thanm 26.5 mcmol/l normally, and may be as sensitive as the bentiromide ^{14}C-PABA test.

p-Aminosalicyclic acid may be used as the marker of absorption instead of ^{14}C-PABA.

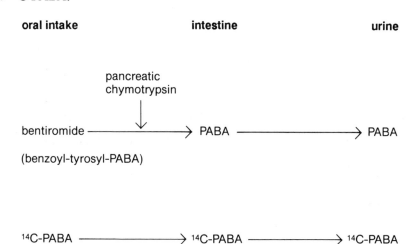

Figure 23 Bentiromide ^{14}C PABA test

References

Mitchell CJ, Field HP, Simpson FG, Parkin A, Kelleher J, Losowsky HS. Preliminary evaluation of a single-day tubeless test of pancreatic function. *Br Med J* 1981; **282**: 1751–3

Tanner AR, Fisher D, Ward C, Smith CL. An evaluation of the one-day NBT-PABA/^{14}C-PABA in the assessment of pancreatic exocrine insufficiency. *Digestion* 1984; **29**: 42–6

Meyer BM, Campbell DR, Curington CW, Toskes PP. Bentiromide test is not affected in patients with small bowel disease or liver disease. *Pancreas* 1987; **2**: 44–7

Delchier J-C, Soule J-C. BT-PABA test with plasma PABA measurements: evaluation of sensitivity and specificity. *Gut* 1983; **24**: 318–25

Weizman Z, Forstner GG, Gaskin KJ, Kopelman H, Wong S, Durie PR. Bentiromide test for assessing pancreatic dysfunction using analysis of PABA in plasma and urine. *Gastroenterology* 1985; **89**: 596–604

Hoek FJ, Van Den Bergh FAJIM, Elhorst JTK, Meijer JC, Timmer E, Tygat GNJ. Improved specificity of the PABA test with PAS. *Gut* 1987; **28**: 468–73

Fluorescein dilaurate test (Figure 24)

This is a 3-day procedure. The fasting patient is given two blue capsules of fluorescein dilaurate (0.5 mmol) with a standard breakfast including at least 500 ml fluid. A further litre of fluid should be taken 3–5 hours later, then normal feeding is resumed. Urine is collected for 10 hours and after hydrolysis of a 0.5 ml aliquot with 4.5 ml 0.1 mol/l NaOH, the sample is incubated for 10 min at 65–70°C, cooled and centrifuged. The supernatant is compared with a water standard by fluorimetry at 492 nm and the % dye excreted calculated from the 10-hour volume of urine.

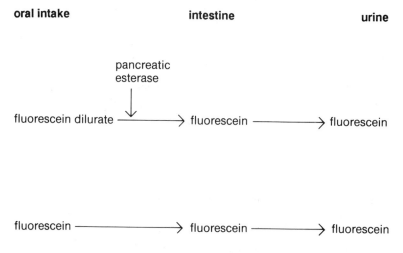

Figure 24 Fluorescein dilaurate test

On the second day after this test the procedure is repeated with one red capsule containing 0.5 mmol fluorescein sodium. The test is then conducted as before.

The ratio of dye excretion after fluorescein dilaurate and after fluorescein sodium should be greater than 0.3. In pancreatic insufficiency the value will be 0.2 or less. Values from 0.2–0.3 are equivocal and the test should be repeated.

An alternative is estimation of serum fluorescein 210 min after oral fluorescein dilaurate 0.5 mmol, which should be 1.5 mcg/ml or more.

The fluorescein dilaurate test can be used in children, where radioactivity should be avoided, but is more tedious to perform despite the ease and reliability of chemical analysis.

References

Lankisch PG, Brauneis J, Otto J, Goke B. Pancreolauryl and NBT-PABA tests. Are serum tests more practicable alternatives to urine tests in the diagnosis of exocrine pancreatic insufficiency? *Gastroenterology* 1986; **90**: 350–4

Barry RE, Barry R, Ene MD, Parker G. Fluorescein dilaurate – tubeless test for pancreatic exocrine failure. *Lancet* 1982; **2**: 742–4

Triolein tests

An oral test of fat absorption using analysis of serum radioactivity after oral ^{14}C-triolein plus ^{3}H-oleic acid has been described. It is also possible to perform a standard ^{14}C-triolein breath test and then repeat it with supplementary pancreatic enzymes, which will normalize breath ^{14}CO$_2$ excretion.

A breath test after oral cholesteryl-^{14}C-octanoate is under evaluation. This depends on pancreatic carboxyl-ester lipase to release ^{14}C-octanoate, which generates ^{14}CO$_2$.

All of these procedures have theoretical attractions, though are not yet standard procedures. The pancreatic-enzyme-supplemented ^{14}C-triolein breath test seems most likely to find a place in diagnosis.

References

Thorsgaard Pedersen N, Marqversen J, Skjoldborg H, Jensen E. Serum radioactivity of ^{14}C-triolein and ^{3}H-oleic acid ingested in a test meal: A rapid test of pancreatic exocrine insufficiency. *Scand J Gastroenterol* 1979; **14**: 529–34

Goff JS. Two-stage triolein breath test differentiates pancreatic insufficiency from other causes of malabsorption. *Gastroenterology* 1982; **83**: 44–6

Cole SG, Stern A, Hofmann AF. Cholesteryl octanoate breath test. *Gastroenterology* 1987; **93**: 1372–80

ORAL GLUCOSE TOLERANCE TEST

This test is described in Chapter 6.

An elevated blood sugar concentration and glycosuria occurs in 15% of patients with *acute pancreatitis*. In *chronic pancreatitis* some abnormality of glucose tolerance occurs in 70% of patients. Glucose tolerance is invariably abnormal in the presence of *pancreatic steatorrhoea*. The test is frequently abnormal when there is derangement of the pancreatic exocrine function tests. Occasionally an abnormal test is the only manifestation of pancreatic disease. Some abnormality of glucose metabolism has been demonstrated in 20–30% of patients with *pancreatic cancer*. It is thought to have an endocrine basis more complex than simple destruction of the beta-cells of the islets.

An *intravenous test* is used to avoid difficulties arising from defective glucose absorption. Such a test is generally unnecessary, because glucose absorption is usually normal in pancreatic disease even when steatorrhoea is present. Occasionally the test is undertaken to test for diabetes mellitus in patients with coeliac disease or after partial gastrectomy.

DIGESTIVE ENZYMES OUTSIDE THE GUT

At least a dozen digestive enzymes are formed by the pancreas. Not all of them are readily measured in the serum and only three, amylase, trypsin and lipase, have been studied clinically to any extent.

Serum amylase

The units of amylase activity vary according to the method and the upper limit of normal is 300–400 iu. The serum amylase may be expressed in international, Somogyi, Lagerlöf or Wohlgemuth units. The methods are potentially less accurate when there is hyperglycaemia and in the presence of jaundice. Lipaemia interferes with the assay, which should be performed only after dilution of the serum by 5–100 times until further dilution produces no more apparent increase in levels.

Interpretation

Characteristically there is elevation of serum amylase concentration in *acute pancreatitis*. The rise starts within 2–12 hours of the inflammation, is maximally elevated by the second to fourth day and falls to normal values within 3–6 days. There is no single blood level which is diagnostic for pancreatitis, but an increase five times the upper limit of normal is regarded as diagnostic of acute pancreatitis and levels over twice normal are suggestive. It is not possible to predict the extent of the pancreatic damage from the serum levels. A fall in serum level does not necessarily indicate any improvement in the disease because it may be the consequence of severe destruction of acinar tissue.

There are a number of *extra-pancreatic* causes of an elevated serum amylase level including perforated peptic ulcer, small bowel obstruction, peritonitis, viral hepatitis, ectopic pregnancy, inflammation of the salivary glands, and uraemia, but they seldom cause a five-fold elevation. Drugs such as morphine and codeine which produce spasm of the sphincter of Oddi may cause a rise in the serum amylase concentration. Therefore, it is always advisable to stop these drugs for at least 24 hours before estimating serum amylase. In all these situations the rise in serum amylase concentration is seldom more than three to four times the normal value.

The serum amylase concentration usually returns to normal within a week and persistent elevation generally implies the development of a *pancreatic pseudocyst*. Less common causes of a prolonged elevation of the serum amylase are persistent pancreatitis, partial pancreatic duct obstruction and renal failure.

Macroamylasaemia is a rare cause of raised levels in which there is binding of the amylase to an abnormal globulin with the formation of a macromolecular complex which is too large to be excreted via the kidneys. This unusual cause is suggested when there is an elevated serum amylase concentration in association with normal or reduced urinary concentrations of the enzyme.

Serum amylase increases usually do not occur in chronic pancreatitis or pancreatic cancer, and if there is elevation it is of a modest degree only. Isoenzyme analysis may be useful to determine the origin of amylase, as in pancreatic insufficiency.

Urinary amylase

Normally amylase is cleared by the kidneys and there is a two to three-fold rise in acute pancreatitis. The excretion of amylase may be used as an index of pancreatic amylase released into the blood.

The test is usually performed on a 24-hour sample of urine collected into a bottle containing toluene. An increased urinary excretion of enzyme occurs in *acute pancreatitis*. Low values are recorded when there is associated renal failure. An estimation can be performed on a single urine sample in an emergency, but this is inaccurate because enzyme values vary according to the degree of concentration of the sample. Urinary amylase has been expressed as the amount excreted per unit of time in an attempt to increase the accuracy of urinary amylase as a diagnostic test. The hourly excretion rate of the enzyme may be abnormal when the serum enzyme levels are normal.

The urinary amylase concentration falls rapidly although it may take longer than the serum levels to return to normal, and may occasionally remain elevated for 1–2 weeks. The urine analysis may, therefore, be used to diagnose acute pancreatitis at a late stage. The test is of no value in the diagnosis of chronic pancreatic disease.

In an attempt to correct for the hyperamylasaemia of renal failure and for the frequent association of renal impairment with acute pancreatitis, the amylase:creatinine clearance ratio has been proposed. This is based on simultaneous estimation in the serum and urine of both amylase and creatinine. It has not proved as helpful as was originally hoped and is not recommended.

Amylase in other fluids

It is often of value to estimate the amylase activity in ascitic and pleural fluid. High values suggest the presence of acute pancreatitis. The elevation may be as high as blood levels and may persist for 2–3 days longer than in serum. This is sometimes of diagnostic value.

Serum lipase

Elevations parallel those of serum amylase though they are more prolonged and uniform. The only added information is gained in abdominal pain with mumps or alcoholic parotitis, because lipase, unlike amylase, is not produced in the salivary glands in appreciable amounts.

Serum trypsin

This is increased in acute pancreatitis, but biological assay is not practicable because of powerful serum antitrypsin activity. Radioimmunoassay has been introduced to obviate this problem. Although theoretically superior to serum amylase estimation because of its greater specificity, serum trypsin measurement has not yet been shown convincingly to confer any practical advantages in adults, despite claims that values over 20 mg/ml trypsin-like immunoreactivity indicate a pancreatic cause in steatorrhoea. However, in infancy dried blood spot assay can be used to screen for cystic fibrosis, where values are usually greater than 80 mg/l.

References

Steinberg WM, Goldstein SS, Davis ND, Shama'a J, Anderson K. Diagnostic assays in acute pancreatitis. *Ann Intern Med* 1985; **102**: 576–80

Salt WB, Schenker S. Amylase – its clinical significance: A review of the literature. *Medicine* 1967; **55**: 269–89

Elias E, Redshaw M, Wood T. Diagnostic importance of changes in circulating concentration of immunoreactive trypsin. *Lancet* 1977; **2**: 66–8

Jacobson DG, Curington C, Connery K, Toskes PP. Trypsin-like immunoreactivity as a test for pancreatic insufficiency. *N Engl J Med* 1984; **310**: 1307–9

Crossley JR, Elliott RB, Smith PA. Dried blood–spot screening for cystic fibrosis in the newborn. *Lancet* 1979; **i**: 472–4

Heeley AF, Heeley ME, King DN, Kuzemko JA, Walsh MP. Screening for cystic fibrosis by dried blood spot trypsin assay. *Arch Dis Child* 1982; **57**: 18–21

Nasrallah SM, Martin DM. Serum isoamylase as a test for pancreatic insufficiency. *Gut* 1983; **24**: 161–4

Junglee D, Penketh A, Katrak A, Hodson ME, Batten JC, Dandona P. Serum pancreatic lipase activity in cystic fibrosis. *Br Med J* 1983; **286**: 1693–4

OTHER BLOOD TESTS

Serum calcium

Normal levels are 2.15–2.65 mmol/l when serum albumin is 40 g/l. A correction can be made for reduced albumin levels by multiplying the number of g/l under 40 g/l by 0.2, and adding the results to the estimated value. Thus, an apparent serum calcium of 2.09 mmol/l with an albumin of 31 g/l corrects to 2.27 mmol/l. A similar correction can be made for elevated serum albumin levels by multiplying the number of g/l over 40 g/l by 0.02 mmol/l and subtracting the result from the apparent serum calcium.

The serum calcium level is commonly reduced during an attack of acute pancreatitis. It is important to correct values for serum albumin levels, which are often also markedly reduced. The maximum fall in serum calcium is seen 1–2 days after the onset of the attack of pancreatitis. A normal or elevated serum calcium level in the presence of severe pancreatic inflammation should raise the suspicion of associated hyperparathyroidism.

Serum bilirubin

The serum bilirubin may be elevated during an attack of acute pancreatitis. The presence of an elevated value in a patient with recurrent or chronic pancreatitis should always raise the suspicion of pancreatic cancer, though it is not pathognomonic.

Serum alkaline phosphatase

An elevation of serum alkaline phosphatase may be found when there is duct obstruction as might occur in pancreatic cancer. Isolated raised alkaline phosphatase levels also occur in liver metastases. The association of bone disease with pancreatic dysfunction may be responsible for raised alkaline phosphatase values and this occurs when there is chronic pancreatic insufficiency and steatorrhoea, or hyperparathyroidism and pancreatitis.

Blood gases

In acute pancreatitis there are frequently various disturbances of pulmonary function, and reduction in the arterial oxygen tension (PaO_2) is one of the most constant findings in the condition.

STOOL EXAMINATION

Macroscopic and microscopic examination

In pancreatic insufficiency the stool may appear normal or it may show obvious steatorrhoea by being pale, bulky and offensive.

The stool can be examined for fat droplets and meat fibres. Normally not more than one or two partially digested meat fibres are seen in a high-power field. The fibres are free from striations and have rounded ends but no nuclei. In pancreatic insufficiency there may be an increase in the number of meat fibres and they are partially digested with striations, irregular ends, and nuclei.

Gallstones can be found in the stools of patients with gallstone pancreatitis.

Steatorrhoea

Steatorrhoea may occur during an episode of acute pancreatitis, the stool fat output frequently returning to normal once the inflammation has subsided. Excess fat in the stool may be a prominent feature of chronic pancreatitis and is found in up to 50% of patients. Steatorrhoea is seldom the sole manifestation of pancreatic disease. Fat maldigestion is even less common in pancreatic cancer, occurring in under 20% of patients. It is most likely to occur in cancer of the head of the pancreas.

149

Stool trypsin and chymotrypsin

These may be estimated in a number of ways.

Faecal chymotrypsin measurement in adults is a less sensitive test for pancreatic insufficiency than duodenal drainage after pancreatic stimulation. By contrast, in children the test can be very reliable as an index of pancreatic function. Analysis of a 3-day stool collection gives values of 2 mg chymotrypsin/kg body weight or less in cystic fibrosis with steatorrhoea, compared with normal values of 3 mg/kg collection.

References

Acosta JM, Ledesma CL. Gallstone migration as a cause of acute pancreatitis. *N Engl J Med* 1974; **290**: 484 – 7

Johnstone DE. Studies of cystic fibrosis of the pancreas. *Am J Dis Child* 1952; **84**: 191 – 8

Haverback B, Dyce BJ, Gutentag PJ, Montgomery DW. Measurement of trypsin and chymotrypsin in stool: A diagnostic test for pancreatic exocrine insufficiency. *Gastroenterology* 1963; **44** 588 – 97

Gordon I, Levin B, Whitehead TP. Estimation of trypsin in duodenal juice. *Br Med J* 1952; i: 463 – 5

Durr HK, Otte M, Forell MM, Bode JC. Faecal chymotrypsin: a study on its diagnostic value by comparison with the secretin-CCK test. *Digestion* 1978; **17**: 404 – 9

Bonin A, Roy CC, Lasalle R, Weber A, Morin CL. Faecal chymotrypsin: a reliable index of exocrine pancreatic function in children. *J Paediatr* 1973; **83**: 594 – 60

SWEAT ELECTROLYTES

The measurement of the sweat electrolyte concentration is an important investigation in the child with steatorrhoea and malabsorption. Children with fibrocystic disease of the pancreas (mucoviscidosis) have a raised concentration of sodium chloride in the sweat. This fundamental abnormality is present regardless of the pancreatic function. The sweat electrolyte excretion is not abnormal in other varieties of pancreatic disease or malabsorption. Pilocarpine iontophoresis is the recommended technique for measuring the sweat electrolyte concentration, but similar results to this test are obtained using methacholine chloride stimulation.

Pilocarpine iontophoresis

Method

Sweat is collected at room temperature from the flexor aspects of either forearm. A direct current source is used. The positive electrode is filled with

0.5% aqueous pilocarpine nitrate solution and the negative with 1% aqueous sodium nitrate solution. The surface of the positive electrode is covered with a circle of ashless filter paper saturated with pilocarpine nitrate solution and the negative electrode with a gauze saturated in the sodium nitrate solution. This is to prevent stinging. A rubber strap holds the positive electrode in place at the midpoint of the flexor surface, and the negative electrode on the extensor surface of the forearm. Circular electrodes are used with a 3 cm diameter.

A current of 1.5 mA is passed for 5 min. The electrodes are removed and 5 min later the area covered by the positive electrode is washed with distilled water and covered with a circle of Whatman No.40 ashless filter paper of known weight. The paper is carefully handled with forceps. It is covered with Parafilm and the sweat collected for 25–35 min. The paper is removed, weighed, placed in a flask and the electrolytes eluted in 10 ml distilled water. The sodium and chloride concentrations are measured by routine methods.

Interpretation

In *normal infants* the mean sweat sodium is 24 mmol/l and chloride 19 mmol/l. In *cystic fibrosis* the mean concentrations are 110 and 117 mmol/l, respectively, and values greater than 70 mmol/l establish the diagnosis. Sweat chloride is the more reliable index.

After the first month of life the sweat sodium and chloride concentrations drop and are low by the end of the first year. Thereafter sweat electrolyte concentration increases with age.

A greater range of normal values is found in adults and levels are found which overlap the fibrocystic range. No sex difference is observed in children, but adult females have lower sweat sodium concentrations than males.

In *adults* the separation of cystic fibrosis from normal is much less satisfactory, but values of sweat electrolytes over 90 mmol/l are suggestive in a single test, or over 70 mmol/l in each of two tests.

Similar results may be obtained by the use of subcutaneous injection of 2 mg methacholine chloride instead of iontophoresis.

Skin chloride assay

This employs the principle of measuring the chloride content of sweat directly on the skin.

First the skin-chloride electrode is calibrated. A pilocarpine-impregnated pad is applied to a well-washed and dried area of the forearm. Current is passed for 5 min, the pad is removed and the area is washed and dried again.

The area is then covered with Parafilm and the presence of sweating is observed. Failure to detect sweating invalidates the test.

The direct-reading skin-chloride electrode is placed on the skin immediately the Parafilm is removed, taking care that good contact is made without trapping air. The chloride concentration is then read directly.

The sweat tests are not infallible and reproducibility can be poor; it is important that they are interpreted with regard to clinical features. Screening of neonatal blood for immunoreactive trypsin, detection of serum cystic-fibrosis protein, estimation of salivary and nail-clipping electrolytes, and screening meconium for albumin have all been proposed for the diagnosis of cystic fibrosis.

References

Gibson LE, Cooke RE. A test for concentration of electrolytes in sweat in cystic fibrosis of the pancreas using pilocarpine by iontophoresis. *Paediatrics* 1959; **23**: 545 – 9
Denning CR, Huang NN, Cuasay LR *et al.* Co-operative study comparing 3 methods of performing sweat tests in cystic fibrosis. *Paediatrics* 1980; **66**: 752 – 7
Bray PT, Clark GCF, Moody GJ, Thomas JDR. Sweat testing for cystic fibrosis: errors associated with the in-situ sweat test using chloride ion selective electrodes. *Clin Chim Acta* 1977; **80**: 333 – 8
Warwick WJ, Hansen L. Measurement of chloride in sweat with the chloride selective electrode. *Clin Chem* 1978; **24**: 2050 – 3
Hodson M, Beldon I, Power R, Duncan FR, Bamber M, Batten JC. Sweat tests to diagnose cystic fibrosis in adults. *Br Med J* 1983; **286**: 1381 – 3

GUT ENDOCRINOLOGY

Many hormones and candidate hormones have been identified in the gastrointestinal tract since the original description of secretin in 1902. Peptides with a known physiological role are secretin, gastrin, cholecystokinin – pancreozymin and glucagon. There are others including vasoactive intestinal peptide (VIP), gastric inhibitary peptide (GIP), motilin, bombesin, substance P, pancreatic polypeptide (PP) and the potent secretion-inhibitor somatostatin. More recently the endorphins and the prostaglandins have been postulated to have important functions. Because the physiological role of most of the hormones is doubtful, measuring levels in tissue and serum does not usually assist in diagnosis, with the important exception of the endocrine tumours or hyperplasias which are frequently located in the pancreatic islets. The two most common of these are insulinomas and gastrinomas (causing the Zollinger-Ellison syndrome). Well-recognized but rare are glucagonomas, and vipomas (causing the watery diarrhoea/hypokalaemia/achlorhydria or Verner – Morrison syndrome from overproduction of vasoactive intestinal peptide).

Insulinoma

This is a notoriously difficult tumour to diagnose. Symptoms can include periodic dizziness and blackouts, epileptic fits and psychiatric disturbances. It is necessary to demonstrate both that the symptoms are due to hypoglycaemia and that the hypoglycaemia is the consequence of an insulin-secreting tumour of the beta-cells of the pancreatic islets.

The diagnosis depends on the demonstration of hypoglycaemia with appropriately high insulin levels.

Prolonged starvation

The patient is fasted for up to 72 hours but allowed to drink water. This induces hypoglycaemia and produces symptoms which are relieved by rapid intravenous glucose administration. The test is carried out in the hospital with careful supervision of the patient. Blood sugar samples are taken at regular intervals (at least twice daily) and also if symptoms develop. Two-thirds of patients with insulinomas develop symptoms within 24 hours and virtually all do so within 48 hours; the demonstrations of a blood glucose of less than 1.7 mmol/l when there are symptoms is especially useful.

At the times of blood sugar estimation, samples of serum are taken and stored frozen. If the patient develops hypoglycaemia then these are analysed for immunoreactive insulin. A positive diagnosis is made by the finding of a ratio of

$$\frac{\text{Immunoreactive insulin (mcU/ml)}}{\text{Blood glucose (mmol/l)}}$$

of 0.3 or greater.

Glucagon test

Glucagon 1 mg is injected intravenously and venous blood samples are taken at 0, 10, 20, 30, 45, 60, 90, 120, 150 and 180 min. An assay is made for glucose and insulin. In normal subjects the blood sugar rises and falls much as in an oral glucose tolerance test. When an insulinoma is present the period of raised blood sugar levels is shorter and is followed by an abrupt and pronounced fall in blood sugar, even to hypoglycaemic levels. Plasma insulin levels are greater than 100 mcmol/ml after 10 min. This is in many respects the safest of the provocative tests.

The test can be performed by injecting 1 mg glucagon intramuscularly and testing the capillary blood.

Tolbutamide test

The patient takes a diet containing 300 g carbohydrate for 3 days before the test. After an overnight fast 1 g tolbutamide is administered intravenously in 20 ml normal saline over 1–2 min. Venous blood samples are taken at 0, 10, 20, 30, 45, 60, 90, 120, 150 and 180 min and assayed for glucose and insulin. The test is positive when the blood glucose fails to return to 66% of the fasting value by 180 min. An early fall in blood glucose is of no diagnostic value.

When an insulinoma is present there is an elevated fasting insulin, the plasma insulin rises to above 120 mcU/ml within 10–30 min, and the insulin level fails to return to normal within 60 min.

This test is unnecessary and dangerous if the fasting blood sugar is below 1.7 mmol/l. Glucose and hydrocortisone must be available during the test. The timing of samples is critical. False-positive results are rare but may occur in liver disease.

L-Leucine test

The patient ingests 150–200 mg L-leucine/kg body weight. The leucine is prepared in a palatable form by the pharmacy without using sugar. Alternatively 200 mg L-leucine/kg body weight is administered intravenously over 10 min. Samples of venous blood are taken at 0, 15, 30, 45, 60 and 90 min and assayed for glucose and insulin. In normal adults there is often a slight fall of blood glucose concentration of up to 1 mmol/l. In an adult the diagnosis of insulinoma is suggested by a fall of blood glucose by more than 1 mmol/l in samples taken at 15, 30, 45 or 60 min. The diagnosis is also suggested by a plasma insulin rise of more than 20 mcU/ml.

This is a useful test for the diagnosis of insulinoma in the adult, but not in children where insulinoma is rare.

Arteriography

This is of great help in the diagnosis of insulinomas. A well-defined round vascular shadow is often seen in the pancreatic substance. The tumours are usually too small to be demonstrated by the more routine radiological procedures or by pancreatic scanning.

Half of the islet cell tumours are not well differentiated. The possibilities of multiple hormone production from a single tumour and of multiple endocrine adenomatosis should be borne in mind.

Gastrinoma (Zollinger – Ellison syndrome)

At present only about one-third are diagnosed preoperatively. Clinical features include multiple unusually sited and recurrent peptic ulcers, diarrhoea and steatorrhoea, diabetes mellitus and occasional skin rashes. The best screening test is the measurement of the ratio of basal acid output to peak acid output, which is usually in excess of 60%. Fasting serum gastrin levels over 50 mcmol/l confirm the diagnosis, and a secretin provocation test can be helpful in doubtful cases, when intravenous injection of secretin 1 unit/kg provokes a rapid rise of >50% in serum gastrin levels.

Barium radiology may be helpful, showing coarse gastric folds, multiple ulcers and a dilated and oedematous duodenum. Selective arteriography may localize a pancreatic islet tumour, though frequently undetectable diffuse gastrin-cell hyperplasia occurs.

Glucagonoma

These present with diabetes mellitus, diarrhoea, anaemia, vulvostomatitis and a characteristic necrolitic migratory erythematous skin rash. Elevated serum glucagon levels are found. The *normal* range of serum glucagon is up to 120 pg/ml and levels in *glucagonoma* patients are usually over 1000 pg/ml.

Vipoma (WDHA or Verner – Morrison syndrome)

The clinical features are watery diarrhoea without steatorrhoea, and weakness. Gastric acid secretion is markedly reduced or absent. Hypokalaemia is present and can be severe. Serum vasoactive intestinal peptide levels are usually over 200 pg/ml, compared with normal values of less than 50 pg/ml.

Gut endocrine tumours are relatively uncommon, and with the exception of insulin and gastrin levels the hormone assays are generally only available in highly specialized centres. Clinical features and the simpler investigations should be used to screen those patients in whom hormone assays may be useful.

Serum pancreatic polypeptide >300 mcmol/l may be a reliable marker for a variety of islet cell tumours, and elevated neuron-specific enolase has also been proposed as a useful test.

In intractable diarrhoeas which are undiagnosable despite exhaustive investigation the estimation of a panel of serum hormones such as calcitonin, vasoactive intestinal peptide and pancreatic polypeptide may occasionally be rewarding. Factitious diarrhoea should be borne in mind. It is more common in medical personnel, and may be diagnosed from the clinical history or from an examination of the bedside locker or medicine chest. Some proprietary laxatives contain phenolphthalein, which can be demonstrated in the stool by dropwise addition of 0.1 mol/l sodium hydroxide. In a positive reaction a purple colour develops in the stool.

Pancreatic cancer

The difficulty of diagnosing exocrine pancreatic cancer has stimulated the development of a host of tumour markers such as CEA, pancreatic oncofetal antigen and monoclonal antibody-based tests for CA19-9 and CA 125.

None is entirely specific or satisfactory, but they may play a role in combination with other tests and in serial monitoring of progress in individuals.

References

Nishida K, Sugira M, Yoshikawa T, Kondo M. Enzyme immunoassay of pancreatic oncofetal antigen (POA). *Gut* 1985; **26**: 450–5

Steinberg WM, Gelfand R, Anderson KK *et al.* Comparison of the sensitivity and specificity of the CA19-9 and CEA assays in detecting cancer of the pancreas. *Gastroenterology* 1986; **90**: 343–9

Sakamoto K, Haga Y, Yoshimura R, Egami H, Yokoyama Y, Akagi M. Comparative effectiveness of the tumour diagnostics CA19-9, CA125 and CEA in patients with diseases of the digestive system. *Gut* 1987; **28**: 323–9

Adrian TE, Uttenthal LO, Williams SJ, Bloom SR. Secretion of pancreatic polypeptide in patients with pancreatic endocrine tumours. *N Engl J Med* 1986; **315**: 287–91

Iwase K, Kato K, Nagasaka H *et al.* Immunohistochemical study of neuron-specific enolase (NSE) and CA19-9 in pancreatic disorders. *Gastroenterology* 1986; **91**: 576–80

Walsh JH, Tomkins RK, Taylor IL, Lechago J, Hansky J. Gastrointestinal hormones in clinical disease: recent developments. *Ann Intern Med* 1979; **90**: 817–28

Adrian TE, Bloom SR, Bryant MG, Polak JM, Heitz PH, Barnes AJ. Distribution and release of human pancreatic polypeptide. *Gut* 1976; **17**: 940–4

Bloom SR, Polak JM. Plasma hormone concentrations in gastrointestinal disease. *Clin Gastroenterol* 1980; **9**: 785–98

Liver biochemistry

Many of the advances in our knowledge about liver disease have followed the wider use of liver biopsy and development of new techniques such as ultrasonography and computed tomography. Nevertheless, blood tests remain the first investigations in the assessment of liver dysfunction. None of the tests is entirely specific, and interpretation usually depends on examination of a constellation of results together with the clinical presentation. There is no true 'liver function test'.

SERUM BILIRUBIN

Although harmless in adults the visible nature of hyperbilirubinaemia makes this an obvious marker of liver disease. Jaundice may, however, result from three distinct processes:

Haemolysis. There is excess production of unconjugated bilirubin due to red cell destruction. The jaundice is usually independent of hepatobiliary disease.

Hepatocellular damage. There is a failure of conjugation of bilirubin, which accumulates in the bloodstream, but some reduction in excretory capacity for conjugated bilirubin may also contribute to the raised serum bilirubin.

Cholestasis. Conjugated bilirubin is not excreted because of dysfunction of the bile secretory mechanism at the bile canaliculus *(intrahepatic choles-tasis)* or because of an *extrahepatic obstruction.*

These causes can be inter-related. For example, cirrhosis with some liver cell necrosis may be accompanied by intrahepatic cholestatis and haemolysis.

Patients with carotenaemia from excess dietary carotene or associated with hypothyroidism may also develop yellow skin, but unlike hyperbilirubin-aemia there is no conjunctival colouring.

Jaundice is usually detectable when serum bilirubin rises above 50 mcmol/l, and can often be seen at lower levels. Variable tissue levels in fluctuating jaundice may mean that skin and conjunctival appearances do not correlate.

Laboratory measurements of serum bilirubin are based on a diazo colour reaction which forms the purple azobilirubin. Conjugated (direct) bilirubin reacts quickly. Unconjugated (indirect) bilirubin reacts slowly and requires the addition of alcohol for complete reaction. There are considerable technical problems associated with fractionation of bilirubin, and at very low levels of total bilirubin, as well as when there is considerable elevation, the ratio of conjugated:unconjugated bilirubin is unreliable. An alternative assay using alkaline methanolysis and high performance liquid chromatography yields lower and different results, which could be useful in assessing the significance of marginal hyperbilirubinaemia.

Interpretation

The normal serum bilirubin is less than 17 mcmol/l in women and less than 23 mcmol/l in men. Half or less is conjugated. In *haemolysis* there is increase in unconjugated bilirubin, and unless there is associated liver disease the conjugated bilirubin level remains low.

In *cholestasis* ('obstructive' jaundice, either intra- or extrahepatic) the conjugated bilirubin is characteristically raised. Prolonged cholestatis may, however, lead to liver failure, and there may also be some elevation of unconjugated bilirubin.

In *hepatocellular damage* both fractions of bilirubin are raised though usually unconjugated bilirubin predominates. Occasionally the rise is due entirely to conjugated bilirubin.

For serial monitoring of the progress of liver disease total bilirubin measurement is adequate.

URINE BILIRUBIN

Conjugated, but not unconjugated bilirubin is excreted in the urine.

URINE UROBILINOGEN

Urobilinogens are formed from bilirubin by bacterial action in the intestine. Most are excreted in the faeces but some are absorbed and excreted in the urine. The excretion is maximal between 2 and 4 p.m. and is enhanced by an alkaline urine. On exposure to air the urobilinogen is oxidized to urobilin, which darkens the urine.

Method

Ehrlich's reagent 1 ml is added to 10 ml freshly voided urine. The Ehrlich's reagent is made up by dissolving 2 g p-dimethylaminobenzaldehyde in 100 ml 20% hydrochloric acid. If much bilirubin is present it is precipitated by adding 10% barium chloride to the urine and the filtrate is tested. -

Interpretation

Normal urine gives either no colour reaction or only a faint red colour which is intensified by gentle heating. A distinctly red colour in the cold is indicative of increased amounts of urobilinogen. A rough quantitation can be made by serial dilutions of the coloured urine to find the greatest dilution which shows a pink colour. Normal urine shows no colour when diluted more than 1:20.

A false-negative result may be given if urine is tested after it has been standing for some time at room temperature. Antibiotic therapy may result in urobilinogen being absent from the urine because of the destruction of the intestinal bacteria. The test is a useful method for distinguishing between obstructive jaundice on the one hand and hepatocellular and haemolytic jaundice on the other. In the former there is no urobilinogen in the urine whereas in the latter conditions urobilirubinogenuria may be present. A positive result can be found in many febrile patients.

Porphobilinogen also forms a red compound with Ehrlich's reagent. To differentiate porphobilinogens from urobilinogens 1 ml saturated sodium acetate and 2 ml chloroform are added to the test tube containing the urine and Ehrlich's reagent. The tube is shaken and the mixture allowed to settle. Urobilinogen dissolves into the lower (chloroform) layer which turns pink but no such change occurs with porphobilinogen which remains in the colourless upper aqueous phase.

Testing for urinary urobilinogen has been simplified by the introduction of a dipstick test which provides a semiquantitative record.

In the presence of cholestasis the stools become pale because of absence of bile pigment in the intestine. This does not occur in haemolysis or hepatocellular jaundice.

SERUM ENZYMES

A number of intracellular enzymes appear in the serum when liver cells are damaged. Different patterns of elevation suggest different disorders, but none is pathognomonic. The mechanism of elevated serum levels is leakage from the cells linked with the increased synthesis of enzymes because of induction prior to necrosis.

Table 2 Changes in bile pigment metabolism associated with the various types of jaundice

| Disease | Stool appearance | Urine | | Appearance | Blood | |
		Urobilinogen	Bilirubin		Conjugated bilirubin	Unconjugated bilirubin
Haemolytic jaundice	Normal	Increased	Absent	Normal	Normal	Increased
Cholestatic jaundice	Pale	Absent	Present	Dark	Increased	Normal or increased
Hepatocellular jaundice	Normal	Variable (high, low, normal)	Present	Normal	Increased	Increased

Transaminases

Both aspartate aminotransferase, EC 2.6.1.1 (AST, SGOT) and alanine aminotransferase, EC 2.6.1.2 (ALT, SGPT) are released in hepatocellular damage. ALT is slightly more specific to the liver.

The normal serum AST concentration is up to 40 iu/l and the normal ALT up to 50 iu/l. Marked elevations in concentration occur in acute hepatitis and hepatic necrosis, and levels of 150–1000 iu/l are fairly common. Lesser elevation, usually below 150 iu/l, are recorded in infectious mononucleosis, drug cholestasis, metastatic cancer of the liver, cirrhosis and extrahepatic obstruction. Occasionally marked elevations of ALT + AST concentration are found in extrahepatic obstruction. On the other hand, patients may die from acute hepatitis without an elevation in serum enzyme concentrations. Thus transaminase levels have their limitations in the diagnosis of liver disease and jaundice. The serum transaminase concentration may be the only biochemical abnormality present in patients with hepatitis and this estimation has been used in epidemiological screening studies.

ALT + AST are present in many of the body cells and elevated serum levels accompany bowel necrosis, pancreatitis, myocardial infarction and other disorders. These conditions are usually readily distinguished from liver disease and, therefore, the source of an elevated level is seldom a problem when investigating a patient with liver disease. In liver disease where the AST is greater than twice the ALT level, alcohol is thought likely to be the cause.

Alkaline phosphatase

The serum alkaline phosphatase EC 3.1.3.1 originates from the liver, bones, intestines and placenta. The upper limit of normal is 100 international units (iu). Children and adolescents normally have increased serum alkaline phosphatase concentration levels because of bone growth.

The serum alkaline phosphatase is a relatively insensitive test of hepatocellular function. The concentration is raised in the presence of intra- or extrahepatic biliary obstruction. A normal value excludes mechanical obstruction of the bile ducts with 95% confidence. A more moderate increase in enzyme levels is found in acute hepatitis and cirrhosis. High levels in a patient with cirrhosis suggest the presence of either co-existent biliary tract disease or a hepatoma. Elevated concentrations in the absence of jaundice may be found in primary and secondary liver tumours, primary biliary cirrhosis, lesions of the bile duct, abscesses, granulomas and amyloidosis. While this enzyme is of help for determining whether there is obstruction to the outflow of bile, or irritation of the biliary epithelium, it is of no value in deciding the site of the lesion.

Elevated serum concentrations are found in bone disorders in which there is increased osteoblastic activity such as Paget's disease, osteogenic secondary deposits, osteomalacia and rickets. The identification and differentiation of the serum alkaline phosphatase isoenzymes is technically difficult. The electrophoretic characteristics of the alkaline phosphatases of skeletal and hepatic origin are similar, but they can be separated on polyacrylamide gel.

Gamma-glutamyl transferase

The test for this enzyme (EC 2.3.2.2) (Gamma-GT) is the most sensitive widely available test of disordered hepatobiliary function. Unfortunately it is non-specific, and the level can be raised in pancreatic and renal disease, as well as by drug induction of liver enzymes.

Normal values are up to 50 iu/l. It is particularly useful in the diagnosis of alcoholic liver disease. Elevated levels are characteristic of biliary disease and all the disorders which raise hepatic alkaline phosphatase levels. Since gamma-GT levels are not raised in bone disease, their estimation may help to elucidate the cause of elevated alkaline phosphatase levels. Measurement of gamma-GT is more useful than of 5-nucleotidase which has been superseded.

Other enzymes

There are other enzymes which are somewhat more specific indicators of liver cell damage but their estimation is seldom a necessity. Serum isocitric dehydrogenase (normal levels 1.0–3.5 iu/l) is an example. The serum beta-glucuronidase activity has been recommended as a biochemical index of liver disease in the anicteric subject. It is of no value when the patient is jaundiced. Glutathione-S-transferase is under evaluation and appears promising.

PROTEINS

Albumin

This is synthesized in the liver. Normal serum values are 35–50 g/l and can be affected by a number of factors. There are elevated values in dehydration and low levels in fluid retention. Serum albumin may fall because of increased loss, especially in the nephrotic syndrome or in protein-losing enteropathy. Reduced synthesis may occur in severe malnutrition, such as kwashiorkor, where there are insufficient dietary essential amino acids. Congenitally low levels of albumin occur in $alpha_1$-antitrypsin deficiency, which can cause neonatal hepatitis, cirrhosis and emphysema.

The level of serum albumin is helpful in assessing the severity of liver cell failure as well as in predicting the likely cause of ascites. It should always be available to assist the interpretation of serum calcium levels.

Globulins

Many laboratories report globulin levels as the difference between serum total protein and serum albumin. This is only of very limited usefulness. Much more information is gained by the performance of paper immunoglobulin electrophoresis or by quantitation of serum immunoglobulins.

Immunoglobulins

The normal values for the major immunoglobulins are:

IgG   7–18 g/l
IgA   0.5–4.5 g/l
IgM   0.3–2.5 g/l

The pattern of immunoglobulins is rarely diagnostic and may be affected by diseases which do not involve the gastrointestinal system. There is often considerable overlap in abnormal levels between diseases.

IgG levels are elevated in acute infections including viral hepatitis, and also in chronic active hepatitis; they are reduced in hypogammaglobulinaemia.

IgM levels are elevated in primary biliary cirrhosis and macroglobulinaemia.

IgA levels may be high in cirrhosis. They are usually normal in coeliac disease, and about 1 in 70 patients has low levels. If they are elevated in a patient with coeliac disease then the presence of a lymphoma should be suspected.

Measurement of *IgE* levels (normal up to 100 u/l) may prove of value in appraisal of allergic symptoms.

Electrophoresis

This may provide further information. In myeloma there is a distinct monoclonal band in the gamma-globulins which accounts for the elevated IgG levels. A diffuse increase in gamma-globulins is seen in viral hepatitis and may also occur in cirrhosis. By contrast, an increase in alpha$_2$- and beta-globulins is more characteristic of cholestasis. Alpha$_1$-globulin is markedly reduced or absent in Alpha$_1$-antitrypsin deficiency and in neonatal hepatitis.

References

Killenberg PF, Stevens RD, Wilderman RF, Wilderman NM. The laboratory method as a variable in the interpretation of serum bilirubin fractionisation. *Gastroenterology* 1980; **78**: 1011–5

Skillen AW, Fifield RD, Sheraidah GS. Serum alkaline phosphatase isoenzyme patterns in disease. *Clin Chim Acta* 1972; **40**: 21–5

Burrows S, Feldman W, McBride F. Serum gamma-glutamyl transpeptidase. *Am J Clin Pathol* 1975; **65**: 311–4

Van Wates L, Lieber C. Glutamate dehydrogenase: a reliable marker of liver cell necrosis in the alcoholic. *Br Med J* 1977; **2**: 1508–10

Adachi Y, Horii K, Takahashi Y, Tanahata H, Ohba Y, Yamamoto T. Serum glutathione S-transferase activity in liver diseases. *Clin Chim Acta* 1980; **106**: 243–55

COAGULATION TESTS

Multiple coagulation defects are not uncommon in patients with acute and chronic liver disease. Combined deficiencies of factors II (prothrombin), V, VII and X contribute to an abnormally prolonged prothrombin time. Thus the determination of the one-stage prothrombin time is a useful simple test of liver function. Because vitamin K is a cofactor of hepatic prothrombin synthesis there may be a prolonged prothrombin time in cholestatic jaundice from any cause. The ability of parenteral vitamin K (10 mg vitamin K$_1$ given intramuscularly for 3 days) to convert the prothrombin time to normal values has been used as a diagnostic test for the aetiology of jaundice. Patients with extrahepatic biliary obstruction respond to the vitamin K$_1$ injections, but in severe hepatocellular disease the prothrombin time remains unchanged. This is not a reliable diagnostic test.

Other haematological defects which may be found in liver disease include deficiencies of factors IX (plasma thromboplastin component), XI (plasma thromboplastin antecedent) and platelets.

Liver disease may be accompanied by diffuse intravascular coagulation in which fibrin degradation products appear in the serum (>40 mg/l), the platelet count falls sharply and there is evidence of haemolysis.

BLOOD AMMONIA

Ammonia has been implicated in the genesis of hepatic coma and an estimation of blood ammonia levels may be undertaken in patients with liver disease. Methods for measuring the blood ammonia concentration are complex and are not performed routinely in the management of liver failure. Venous or arterial blood can be sampled and the latter is favoured. The normal arterial blood ammonia concentration is less than 100 mcg/100 ml. Elevated concentrations may be found in hepatocellular failure or when there is shunting of blood from the liver. Arterial blood ammonia levels do not correlate well with the clinical severity of hepatic coma and this correlation is even poorer if venous samples are measured. Elevations of blood ammonia concentration are also found in a variety of rare congenital defects of urea synthesis.

BILE ACIDS

It is possible to measure the concentration of serum bile acids by enzyme fluorimetry, by gas liquid chromatography or by radio-immunoassay. Both total and the major individual bile acids can be accurately quantitated. Normal fasting values are below 4.5 mcmol/l, and postprandial levels less than 6.5 mcmol/l. Elevated values occur in a wide variety of hepatobiliary diseases. Serum bile acids vary with fasting and feeding, during the menstrual cycle, and with vitamin C status in liver disease. There can be a seven-fold fluctuation of values through the day. In addition values may be elevated in small bowel bacterial colonization in hyperlipidaemia, and during bile acid therapy. Serum bile acids are therefore not entirely specific to hepatobiliary disease, and although they can be used for screening and monitoring liver disease they do not add further information to the conventional screen of 'liver function' tests.

Bile acid tolerance tests and clearance studies in which serum levels are measured after oral or intravenous administration of unlabelled or radio-labelled bile acids, give results which are too variable to be helpful in individual diagnosis.

LIPIDS

The normal upper limit for serum cholesterol is 7.8 mmol/l, and for triglycerides is 2.5 mmol/l. Serum total cholesterol rises in both intra- and extrahepatic cholestasis. This results from the presence of an abnormal lipoprotein (LPX) in the serum, which can be measured immunochemically. Very low levels of high-density lipoprotein (HDL) cholesterol are characteristic of cholestasis; the lower limit of normal is about 1 mmol/l.

The presence of altered or abnormal lipoprotein components can be associated with many liver diseases. Raised levels of cholesterol, triglycerides, low-density (LDL)and very low-density (VLDL) lipoproteins in various com-

165

binations is seen. This may be important since markedly elevated serum triglycerides (i.e. $\geqslant$ 10 mmol/l) causes turbidity and interferes with most other biochemical measurements. Alcoholism is the most common cause of secondary hyperlipidaemia, and may itself cause cirrhosis and pancreatitis.

OTHERS

Fluid-electrolyte disturbances including secondary aldosteronism are encountered in liver disease, and *hyponatraemia* (<130 mmol/l) and *hypokalaemia* (<3.5 mmol/l) are common. Although low serum sodium levels are often well tolerated, low serum potassium can potentiate hepatic encephalopathy. *Urea* is synthesized in the liver. Low levels (<3.3 mmol/l) may indicate severe hepatocellular dysfunction but can also reflect dilution with fluid retention. In the presence of associated renal impairment, blood urea may be apparently normal in liver disease, and serum *creatinine* (normal range 45–150 mcmol/l) is a better index of renal failure.

Vitamin B$_{12}$ is normally present in liver cells and levels are elevated in metastatic liver disease, liver abscess and hepatitis. Levels also rise in patients on hydroxocobalamin therapy. Plasma *glucose* levels may be informative as both diabetes mellitus and hypoglycaemia occur in liver disease.

References

Ferraris R, Fiorentini MT, Galatola G, Rolfo P, De la Pierre M. Diagnostic value of serum immunoreactive conjugated cholic or chenodeoxycholic acids in detecting hepato-biliary diseases: comparison with levels of 3 alpha-hydroxy bile acids determined enzymatically and with routine liver tests. *Dig Dis Sci* 1987; **32**: 817–23

Yamanishi Y, Kishimoto Y, Kawasaki H, Hirayama C, Ikawa S. Oral ursodeoxycholic acid tolerance test in patients with digestive disease. *Gastroenterol Jpn* 1981; **16**: 472–7

Mannes GA, Thieme C, Stellard F, Wang T, Sauerbruck T, Paumgartner G. The prognostic significance of serum bile acids in cirrhosis. *Hepatology* 1986; **6**: 50–3

Luey KL, Heaton KW. Bile acid clearance in liver disease. *Gut* 1979; **20**: 1083–7

Engelking LR, Dasher CA, Hirschowitz BI. Within-day fluctuation in serum bile-acid concentration among normal control subjects and patients with hepatic disease. *Am J Clin Pathol* 1980; **73**: 196–201

ALCOHOLIC LIVER DISEASE

Alcohol is the commonest cause of liver disease. The main hurdle in diagnosis is to suspect the cause, and the patient's general demeanour may give clues.

The 'CAGE' questionnaire is a simple 4-point system to assess alcohol abuse. A patient who answers 'yes' to all four questions is an alcoholic, and two to three out of four is suspicious.

(1)   Have you ever tried to Cut down alcoholic intake?

(2)   Have you ever been Annoyed by criticism of your drinking?

(3)   Have you ever felt Guilty about the amount you drink?

(4)   Do you ever take an Eyeopener – a drink to start the day?

Patients may be teetotal at a time when they are suffering the effects of previous heavy drinking, and an assessment of the amount drunk needs to take into account changing patterns.

Patients are not always honest about excess alcohol intake, and laboratory tests are often valuable in establishing diagnoses. They are not infallible, and all can be normal in severe alcoholic liver disease. In addition, a significant minority of alcohol abusers have liver disease for unconnected reasons.

Measurement of the actual level of alcohol in the blood is extremely useful. If there is any alcohol at all in a morning sample then the patient is probably drinking to excess. If the blood alcohol is above 80 mg/dl (the legal limit for driving) at any time during the day, the diagnosis of alcohol excess is likely.

The assessment of long-term heavy drinking is helped by various tests. The most useful are raised gamma GT levels (over 50 u/l) and mean corpuscular volumes (over 95 fl). The alkaline phosphatase level may also be raised to a lesser extent, and the platelet count reduced. Chest radiology may reveal old or recent rib fractures in binge drinkers. Specialized enzyme tests such as glutamate dehydrogenase and mitochondrial AST may prove useful in future but are not generally available.

References

Scharshmidt BF, Blankaert N, Farina FA, Kabra PM, StaffordBE, Weisiger RA.. Measurement of serum bilirubin and its mono- and diconjugates: applicability to patients with hepatobiliary disease. *Gut* 1982; **23**: 643 – 9

Coken JA, Kaplan MM. The SGOT/SGPT ratio – an indicator of alcoholic liver disease. *Dig Dis Sci* 1979; **24**: 835 – 8

Chalmers DM, Rinsler MG, MacDermott S, Spicer CC, Levi AJ. Biochemical and haematological indicators of excessive alcohol consumption. *Gut* 1981; **22**: 992 – 6

Nalpas B, Vassault A, Charpin S, Lacour B, Berthelot P. Serum mitochondrial (m) AST as a marker of chronic alcoholism: diagnostic volume and interpretation in a liver unit. *Hepatology* 1986; **4**: 608 – 14

Penn R, Worthington DJ. Is serum gamma-glutamyltransferase a misleading test? *Br Med J* 1983; **286**: 531 – 5

Skinner HA, Holt S, Sheu WJ, Israel Y. Clinical versus laboratory detection of alcohol abuse: the alcohol clinical index. *Br Med J* 1986; **292**: 1703 – 8

Solberg HE, Skrede S, Blomhoff JP. Diagnosis of liver diseases by laboratory results and discriminant analysis. *Scand J Clin Lab Invest* 1975; **35**: 713 – 21

IMMUNOLOGY

Useful *in vivo* migration and transformation tests may be performed by culture and challenge of lymphocytes with drugs suspected of causing toxic reactions. These should be considered if a patient has had a serious drug reaction, because they may establish the diagnosis without the need for potentially hazardous *in vivo* challenge tests. The peripheral T-cell population is reduced in alcoholic liver disease, chronic acute hepatitis and primary biliary cirrhosis. The human leukocyte antigens HLA-B40 and HLA-B8 are said to be more frequent in patients with alcoholic cirrhosis, compared with other alcoholics and other cirrhotics.

Tumour antigens

Alpha-fetoprotein

This may be detected in the serum of patients with hepatoma (primary liver cell carcinoma). In some parts of the world almost all hepatoma patients have detectable levels, though in northern Europe and North America the figure is lower. It is a reliable test if strongly positive, but expression of results semi-quantitatively has shown some weakly positive results of uncertain significance. It may also be detected in ascitic fluid. This test is also positive in pregnant women carrying fetuses with spinal malformations and in neonatal hepatitis.

Carcinoembryonic and oncofetal antigens

These markers of colonic and pancreatic carcinomas may have a role in monitoring progress of proved disease, such as detected tumour recurrence and metastasis to the liver and elsewhere.

Tissue antibodies

Circulating antibodies to various tissue components have been described in liver disease. While these antibodies are of great theoretical interest, their detection has limited diagnostic significance. The antibodies are detected by various modifications of the two-layer indirect immunofluorescent technique.

Antimitochondrial antibody (AMA)

These antibodies are found in the sera of 95% of patients with primary biliary cirrhosis. They are rarely present in viral or drug hepatitis. Of great diagnostic value is the finding that these antibodies are rarely present in extrahepatic obstruction and then only in a very low titre. These antibodies provide the most diagnostic help of all the antibody tests.

The M_2 ATPase-associated antigen is even more specific for primary biliary cirrhosis.

Antismooth muscle antibody (SMA)

About one-half of patients with chronic active hepatitis demonstrate the presence of antibodies reactive with smooth muscle. Positive reactions also occur in 30% of patients with primary biliary cirrhosis, 25% of patients with idiopathic cirrhosis, and 15% with alcoholic liver disease.

The patients with chronic active hepatitis have high-titre IgG SMA, which is important because 50–80% of patients with viral hepatitis have transient low-titre IgM SMA. There is evidence that the antibody is directed against actin, and the usefulness of measurement of specific antiactin activity is being investigated.

Antinuclear antibody (ANF)

Antinuclear antibody (or factor) is present in 50% of patients with chronic active hepatitis, where it is an IgG antibody in high titre (greater than 1:80). It also occurs commonly in primary biliary cirrhosis and drug-associated chronic hepatitis. Low titres (<1:10) are of no importance.

The more specific antibody directed against double-stranded DNA is a common accompaniment of all forms of liver disease, and does not assist differential diagnosis.

Other antibodies

Liver membrane antibodies, 'liver-specific protein' and bile canalicular antibodies have all been described but are not helpful in diagnosis.

References

Berg PA, Klein R, Lindenborn-Fotinos J et al. ATP-ase-associated antigen (M2); marker

antigen for serological diagnosis of PBC. *Lancet* 1982; **2**: 1423–6
Doniach D, Walker GJ. Mitochondrial antibodies (AMA). *Gut* 1974; **15**: 664–8
Chen D-S, Sung J-L, Sheu J-C. *et al.* Serum alpha-fetoprotein in the early stage of human hepatocellular carcinoma. *Gastroenterology* 1984; **86**: 1404–9

Viral liver disease

Viral hepatitis is usually diagnosed on clinical grounds supported by appropriate biochemical tests. Electron microscopy and liver biopsy provide further evidence. It should usually be possible to define the exact organism involved by serum immunology.

Serum markers

Hepatitis A. Exposure to virus (HAV) is widespread, and infections are mild. Antibody to the virus (anti-HAV) in the IgG class is frequently present in serum of healthy individuals with immunity. The appearance of IgG anti-HAV in a patient known to have beenpreviously negative is evidence of recent exposure. Better proof is the detection of anti-HAV in the IgM class, which is transient but always present at the onset of jaundice in HAV infection.

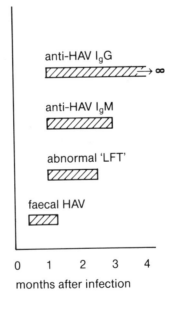

Figure 25 Acute infection with hepatitis A virus (HAV)

Hepatitis B. Acute infection with this virus (HBV) is marked by the appearance in the serum of an antigen associated with the surface protein coat (HB$_s$Ag). It is usually cleared in a matter of weeks, with a rise in a specific antibody directed against it (anti-HB$_s$). In 5–10% of patients HB$_s$Ag persists indefinitely. AntiHB$_s$ is detectable in the serum for long periods and possibly permanently: it only indicates exposure to HBV or surface antigen in vaccine at some time in the past and is not a reliable marker of infectivity.

In acute infection with HBV, antigen from the viral core (HB$_c$ Ag) may sometimes be found in the serum. Antibody to HB$_c$Ag (anti-HB$_c$) is much more commonly found, and the presence of anti-HB$_c$ of the IgM class in high titre reliably indicates recent infection. Another antibody directed against the intact virion may also be found in serum of currently infected patients, as may viral DNA polymerase.

There are other useful markers of HBV infection. In an individual who is a chronic carrier of HB$_s$Ag, the presence of another antigen from the protein coat (HB$_e$Ag) is an indicator of infectivity. If there is antibody to HB$_e$Ag (anti-HB$_e$), or if neither HB$_e$Ag nor anti-HB$_e$ are present, the serum is unlikely to be infectious

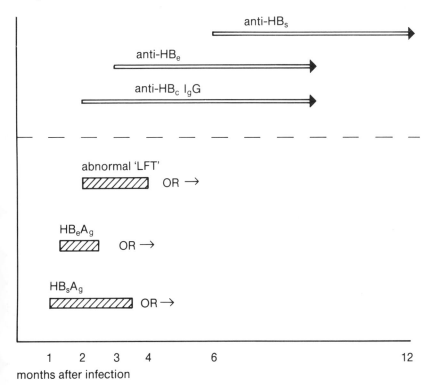

anti-HB$_s$

anti-HB$_e$

anti-HB$_c$ IgG

abnormal 'LFT'
OR →

HB$_e$A$_g$
OR →

HB$_s$A$_g$
OR →

| 1 | 2 | 3 | 4 | 6 | 12 |

months after infection

Figure 26 Acute infection with hepatitis B virus (HBV)

Electron microscopy

The 29 nm particles of the HAV may be found in the stools in acute hepatitis A. The 40–44 nm particles of the HBV are present in the serum of acute hepatitis B, together with spherical and cylindrical remnants of the protein coat.

Liver biopsy

This is often diagnostic, but is not usually necessary to confirm viral hepatitis. It may be misleading early in the illness. Characteristic changes include cloudy swelling of the cytoplasm ('ground-glass' appearance), with the appearance of eosinophilic cell debris (Councilman bodies) and necrotic nuclei.

Immunofluorescence demonstrates intracellular viral antigens, and viral particles can be seen on electron microscopy.

Non-A Non-B hepatitis

An antibody to this virus group has been described. Its reliability is not yet fully established. An indirect test is the absence of elevated transaminase and of HB_s Ag.

Interpretation

Acute HAV infection:

    (1)   presence of IgM class anti-HAV
    (2)   new appearance of IgG class anti-HAV
    (3)   29 nm particles in stool.

Acute HBV infection:

    (1)   new appearance of HB_s Ag or anti-HB_s
    (2)   presence of IgM class anti-HB_c
    (3)   presence of antibody to intact virion or of viral DNA polymerase
    (4)   40–44 nm particles and protein coat remnants in serum.

Chronic HBV infection and carrier state. Any of the markers of HBV infection may be present, with the exception of IgM class anti-HB_c.

Delta viral hepatitis

This RNA virus only affects patients with hepatitis B infection, but may be important in enhancing the pathogenicity of the DNA virus.

In patients positive for HB$_s$Ag the additional presence of IgM anti-delta antibody indicates acute or chronic delta virus infection and may be associated with more severe chronic liver disease. IgG anti-delta antibody merely suggests past infection.

It is also possible to identify delta RNA in the serum and a delta antigen (HD) in serum and liver, but these tests are not generally available.

Table 3 Viral hepatitis markers and their significance

Finding	Usual significance
Hepatitis A:	
IgM anti-HAV	Acute hepatitis A
IgG anti-HAV	Immune to hepatitis A
Hepatitis B:	
HB Ag	Acute or chronic hepatitis B carriage
IgM anti-HB$_c$	Acute hepatitis B (high titre)
	Chronic hepatitis B (low titre)
IgG anti-HB$_c$	Past exposure to hepatitis B (with negative HB$_s$Ag)
	Chronic hepatitis B (with positive HB$_s$Ag)
Anti-HB$_s$	Immune to hepatitis B
HB$_e$Ag	Acute hepatitis B. Persistence means continued infectious state
Anti-HB	Convalescence or continued infectious state
HBV DNA	Continued infectious state
Delta hepatitis:	
IgM anti-delta	Acute infection with delta agent
	Chronic delta infection (high titre)
IgG anti-delta	Past delta infection

Viral hepatitis prevalence

In Britain hepatitis A is the commonest problem. Hepatitis B and delta are decidedly uncommon and afflict mainly risk groups like male homosexuals and i.v. drug addicts. Hepatitis non-A non-B is said to be the commonest cause of post-transfusion viral hepatitis, though this seems to be rare because of the screened voluntary donor system. Transfusion may also spread or reactivate cytomegalovirus, detectable by CMV antibodies.

The pattern is quite different in other countries, and hepatitis B virus-associated hepatoma is said to be the commonest cause of male cancer death worldwide.

References

Lavarini C, Farci P, Chiaberge E, Veglio V, Giacobbi D, Bedarida G, Susani G, Toti M, Almi P, Caporaso N, Del Vecchio Blanco C, Rizzetto M. IgM antibody against hepatitis B core antigen (IgM anti-HBc): diagnostic and prognostic significance in acute HBsAg positive hepatitis. *Br Med J* 1983; **287**: 1254–6

Blum HE, Haase AT, Vyas GN. Molecular pathogenesis of hepatitis B virus infection: simultaneous detection of viral DNA and antigens in paraffin-embedded liver sections. *Lancet* 1984; 771–4

Wantzin P, Nielsen JO, Tygstrup N, Soerensen H, Dybkjaer E. Screening of Danish blood donors for hepatitis B surface antigen using a third generation technique. *Br Med J* 1985; **291**: 780–2

Hoofnagle JH. Type D hepatitis and the hepatitis delta antigen. In Thomas HC, Jones EA (eds.) *Recent Advances in Hepatology* 1986, Edinburgh: Churchill Livingstone, pp. 73–92

Colombo M, Cambieri R, Rumi MG, Ronchi G, Del Ninno E, De Franchis R. Longterm delta superinfection in HBsAg carriers and its relationship to the course of chronic hepatitis. *Gastroenterology* 1983; **85**: 235–9

Fagan EA, Williams R. Serological responses to HBV infection. *Gut* 1986; **27**: 858–67

Lindsay KL, Nizze JA, Koretz R, Gitnick E. Diagnostic usefulness of testing for anti-HB$_c$ IgM in acute hepatitis B. *Hepatology* 1986; **6**: 1325–8

Arico S, Aragona M, Rizzetto M *et al.* Clinical significance of antibody to the hepatitis delta virus in symptomless HBsAg carriers. *Lancet* 1985; **2**: 356–8

Aragona M, Caredda F, Lavarini C, Farci P, Macagno S, Crivelli O, Maran E, Purcell RH, Rizzetto M. Serological response to the hepatitis delta virus in hepatitis D. *Lancet* 1987; **1**: 478–80

Tabor E. The three viruses of non-A, non-B hepatitis. *Lancet* 1985; **1**: 743–5

KINETIC TESTS

Bromsulphthalein (sulphobromophthalein, BSP) retention test

This has been used since 1925. Most of the investigations now used in liver disease have been introduced since then and consequently have tended to replace this investigation. It is used in assessment of anicteric liver disease.

Method

The patient should not be fasting; prolonged fasting alters results. An intravenous injection is given of 5 mg BSP/kg body weight. After 5 and 45 min, 10 ml venous blood is collected from a different vein into a plain test tube and analysed for BSP. The time of collection of the samples is noted accurately.

The injection of BSP may cause allergic reactions such as fever, urticaria and other skin eruptions. Sudden death has occurred. The material is highly irritant and great care must be exercised to avoid extravascular spilling during the injection.

Interpretation

The normal liver clears 95% of the dye within 45 min and less than 0.5 mg/100 ml should remain in the circulation. Thus in normal adults the 45-min BSP retention should not be more than 5%.

A modification of the BSP excretion test is of help in the diagnosis of the *Dubin–Johnson and Rotor syndromes*. Venous blood is collected at 30, 45 and 90 min. The serum BSP concentrations fall at 30 and 45 min and then show a rise at 90 min because of the regurgitation of conjugated BSP into the blood.

The BSP test has been revived somewhat by the introduction of 'compartmented' tests in which serial blood samples are used to calculate disappearance kinetics. The information obtained is usually available by other methods.

Indocyanine green clearance (ICG)

This dye has a number of properties which make it an attractive alternative to BSP. It is relatively free of side-effects; it is avidly taken up and excreted by the liver without conjugation; it is easily measured spectrophotometrically; and this test can be performed at the ear lobe without skin puncture if desired.

Method

An indwelling intravenous cannula is positioned in an arm, and 4 ml blood taken before commencing the test. Ampoules of 2.5% solution of ICG in propandiol are prepared by dilution with four volumes of distilled water (i.e. 1 ml plus 4 ml); 0.3 mg/kg ICG are injected intravenously into the other arm within 30 sec. Five millilitres of blood is taken 2, 4, 6, 8 and 10 min after dye injection, washing the cannula with isotonic saline each time to avoid contamination. The clotted blood sample is centrifuged and the extinction at 814 nm is measured spectrophotometrically using control serum as a blank.

Interpretation

Normal controls have <9% retention at 4 min and <5% retention at 10 min. By contrast patients with liver disease usually retain more than 50% of the initial dose at 4 min, with a mean ICG half-litre of 5–10 min. It can be used as a test of liver blood flow as well as liver cell function.

Aminopyrine breath test

The test is based on the ability of the liver to metabolize ^{14}C-aminopyrine to ^{14}CO$_2$. This metabolism is impaired in severe liver disease.

Method

The fasting patient is given 2 mcCi ^{14}C-aminopyrine orally. Two hours later the amount of ^{14}CO$_2$ trapped in 2 mmol hyamine is measured by liquid scintillation counting. Breath is collected by bubbling through hyamine as for the bile acid breath test (Chapter 7).

Interpretation

Normal subjects excrete 6–12% of the administered dose of ^{14}C in 2 hours. Patients with chronic active hepatitis (CAH) with cirrhosis excrete 2.0% in 2 hours. In alcoholic cirrhosis excretion is 5.5% with some overlap with normals. By contrast, CAH without cirrhosis is associated with normal breath secretion (more than 5%) at 2 hours, and increased excretion is seen in non-cirrhotic alcoholism and with enzyme-inducing drugs.

Ammonia tolerance test

Although fasting venous blood ammonia levels are usually increased in cirrhosis from the normal of 10–35 mcg/100 ml this does not correlate with disease severity nor with encephalopathy.

Method

After an overnight fast an arterial catheter is positioned in the brachial artery. Ammonium chloride 45/mg/kg body weight, up to a maximum of 3 g, is given by mouth. A sample of blood is drawn at 45 min into a heparinized syringe.

Alternative procedures include using ammonium acetate 70 mg/kg or 5–10 g ammonium citrate. Ammonia preparations cause nausea and may be vomited, so rectal administration of ammonium acetate may be used.

Interpretation

Normal subjects have a mean blood ammonia of 117 ± 13 mcg/100 ml at 45 min. In cirrhosis with venous collaterals the mean level is 243 ± 129 mcg/100 ml, but there is a wide overlap with normal. There is also an increase in levels of ammonia in cirrhosis without collateral circulation, and the ammonia tolerance test does not prove that portasystemic shunts are present.

References

Javitt NB. Clinical and experimental aspects of sulphobromophthalein and related compounds. *Progr Liver Dis* 1970; **3**: 110–7

Brügmann E, Towe J. Indocyanine green clearance in a liver function test. *Mater Med Pol* 1974; **6**: 123–6

Grace ND, Castell DO, Wennar MH. A comparison of the oral fructose and ammonia tolerance tests in cirrhosis. *Arch Int Med* 1969; **124**: 330–6

Murew J, Kierulf P. The intravenous galactose test as indication of the extent of fibrosis in patients with cirrhosis of the liver. *Scand J Gastroenterol* 1969; **4**: 453–6

Lewis KO, Nicholson G, Lance P, Paton A. Aminopyrine breath test in alcoholic liver disease and in patients on enzyme inducing drugs. *J Clin Pathol* 1977; **30**: 1040–3

Saunders JB, Lewis KO, Paton A. Early diagnosis of alcoholic cirrhosis by the aminopyrine breath test. *Gastroenterology* 1980; **79**: 112–4

Felding RH, Christensen RF, Lindahl F. Ammonia tolerance test. *Scand J Gastroenterol* 1984; **19**: 365–8

Protein load test

The ability of a cirrhotic patient to tolerate protein in the diet is a guide to the degree of collateral circulation and liver cell function. A diet of increasing amounts of protein is fed while a careful watch is kept on the patient's clinical condition. The starting content of protein in the diet depends on each patient and is usually 40–60 g/day. The patient is observed for the features of impending liver coma which include hepatic foetor, a flapping tremor, slurred speech and drowsiness or restlessness. An electroencephalographic assessment may be made in addition. If no ill-effects are observed after 3 days the protein content of the diet is increased by 20 g/day until 120 g protein/day is reached.

Patients with little shunting of portal blood from the liver and/or good liver function tolerate 120 g protein/day. Patients with sensitivity to protein are unable to tolerate 40 or 60 g protein/day. The test is of value in the selection of patients with portal hypertension for shunt surgery. Those patients with a reduced protein tolerance are expected to do poorly after the operation and are rejected for shunt operations.

ELECTROENCEPHALOGRAPHY (EEG)

The EEG is a useful method for assessing hepatic precoma and coma. The essential change is a progressive slowing of the frequency until the EEG becomes 'delta dominant' and the rhythmic activity is less than 4 cycles/sec. These changes are not specific for liver disease and are found in a number of metabolic confusional states. The prognosis in hepatic failure can be predicted from serial EEGs, prothrombin times and possibly also alpha-feto-protein levels.

CONSTITUTIONAL UNCONJUGATED HYPERBILIRUBINAEMIA (Gilbert's syndrome)

Patients with this condition usually have elevated serum unconjugated and total bilirubin levels, or a history of jaundice in the absence of any other symptoms, or abnormal tests. It is important to make a positive diagnosis in order to allay anxiety about more serious conditions.

Reduced caloric intake test

The patient has blood withdrawn for a total and fractionated serum bilirubin estimation, while taking a normal diet. A diet reduced in energy intake to 1.7 mJ (400 Cal) daily is then given for 2 days and further blood samples are taken at 24 and 48 hours for bilirubin estimation.

A positive result is a rise in serum bilirubin of 100% or more, with the proviso that the rise must be into the abnormal range and be mainly accounted for by an increase in unconjugated bilirubin. Though the test is specific is does not identify all patients; and furthermore individuals with Gilbert's syndrome may have other hepatobiliary disorders. The test depends on appropriate dietetic advice (the permitted daily food intake is equivalent to a modest breakfast), and if this is not available, putting a patient on water only for 2 days can be used.

Other tests that have been used include the administration of nicotinic acid to provoke hyperbilirubinaemia and the infusion of bilirubin followed by serial measurements of serum levels; neither confers any advantage over caloric restriction. It is possible to measure glucuronyl transferase activity in fresh liver biopsy specimen; this is markedly reduced in many, but not all, patients with Gilbert's syndrome, but the test is not widely available.

References

Owens D, Sherlock S. The diagnosis of Gilbert's syndrome: Role of the reduced calorie intake test. *Br Med J* 1973; 3: 559–63

Felsher BF, Carpoi NM. Calorie intake in unconjugated hyperbilirubinaemia. *Gastroenterology* 1975; **69**: 42–7

IDIOPATHIC HAEMOCHROMATOSIS

This diagnosis should only be made when there is no overt cause for iron overload. A strong family history, presence of cardiac and endocrine disease, and absence of alcoholism are valuable pointers.

Serum iron and iron-binding capacity

The normal serum iron is less than 170 mcg/100 ml (or 30 mcmol/l): the average levels are lower in women than men. The average iron binding capacity is 330 mcg/100 ml, with a saturation of 30–40%. Serum iron may fluctuate and is low in many acute and inflammatory diseases.

In haemochromatosis the serum iron is usually raised with a normal iron binding capacity which is 80–100% saturated.

Iron excretion

A simple test, suitable for outpatients, is the measurement of the iron content in a 24-hour urine collection after 0.5 g desferrioxamine intramuscularly. An iron output greater than 36 mcmol (2 mg) indicates iron overload, and in untreated haemochromatosis the excretion is usually over 180 mcmol (10 mg) in 24 hours.

Liver biopsy

This is essential to prove the diagnosis. Iron deposits stain brown with haematoxylin and cosin, and blue with Perl's reagent. In haemochromatosis iron content is + + or more on the semiquantitive 0– + + + + score, and is in excess of 180 mcmol/g (1 g/100 g) dry weight of liver.

Other tests

Excess iron in the reticuloendothelial bone marrow cells occurs and deposits also occur in the skin and gastric mucosa. Serum ferritin levels correlate partially with body iron stores and are usually over 1000 ng/ml in haemochromatosis; this is a very useful screening test for pre-cirrhotic disease.

Liver iron stores are shown as diffuse sonodense areas on ultrasonography and this can be used to monitor removal by treatment.

Patients are usually diabetic, though glucose tolerance is also often impaired in other forms of cirrhosis. The ECG may show dysrhythmias and flattened T waves. Iron absorption is increased (as it is also in porphyria), though this may not be a constant abnormality. Testosterone levels are low and there may be evidence of both adrenal and pituitary failure.

References

Halliday JW, Russo A, Collishaw J, Powell LW. Serum ferritin in the diagnosis of early haemochromatosis: A study of 43 families. *Lancet* 1977; **2**: 621–3
Finch CA, Huebers H. Perspectives in iron metabolism. *N Engl J Med* 1982; **306**: 1520–9

WILSON'S DISEASE

Wilson's disease (hepatolenticular degeneration) is an autosomal recessive disease in which excessive tissue copper deposits occur. It may show itself as nerve damage (Parkinsonism and mental changes) or as liver disease (cirrhosis). Detection of asymptomatic sufferers is important to prevent progression of the disease. Abnormal hepatic copper deposits have been described in other diseases, such as primary biliary cirrhosis, sclerosing cholangitis and chronic cholestasis.

Serum copper and caeruloplasmin

In normal subjects caeruloplasmin levels are 200–400 mg/l. This copper-binding protein with oxidase activity binds 60–120 mcg/100 ml copper in the serum. There is an additional 5–10 mcg/100 ml non-caeruloplasmin copper.

In 95% of patients with Wilson's disease the serum caeruloplasmin levels are belwo 200 mg/l with a serum caeruloplasmin copper under 60 mcg/100 ml. Sometimes the non-caeruloplasmin copper increases in Wilson's disease.

A screening test for copper oxidase activity, taken as equivalent to caeruloplasmin, is widely used. The normal range is 0.2–0.7 optical density units.

Urine copper

The normal subject excretes about 30 mcg/24 hours. In symptomatic Wilson's disease more than 100 mcg/24 hours is excreted, derived from the non-caeruloplasmin serum copper.

Liver biopsy

Cirrhosis is seen and copper can be stained brown-black with rubeanic acid in 70% alcohol. The copper content of the biopsy is measured. In normals this is 20–50 mcg/g dry weight of liver. In Wilson's disease before treatment, liver copper is 250–300 mcg/g dry weight. The biopsy needle must be rendered copper-free by washing with 0.5% EDTA and then rinsing with 5% dextrose.

Kayser – Fleischer rings

These are caused by copper deposits in the cornea. If not obvious to the naked eye they should be sought by slit-lamp examination. They may occur in other causes of copper overload.

HYDATID DISEASE OF THE LIVER

Intradermal (Casoni) test

An intradermal injection of 0.15 ml of hydatid fluid is given into the forearm and a similar volume of sterile normal saline is injected as a control into the other arm. There are two possible positive responses:

(1)   an *immediate* reaction in which a weal appears within 10 min. The maximum diameter, which should be at least 20 mm, is reached within 30 min.

(2)   a *delayed* response which appears after 6 hours and lasts up to 24 hours; this reaction is found less frequently.

A positive test suggests the presence of hydatid disease and is said to occur in

90% of patients with the disease. The test does not satisfactorily distinguish between living and dead cysts. The effectiveness of the antigenic response is liable to variation. False-positive reactions occur in patients who have harboured other types of tapeworm or who are infected with nematodes or trematodes.

A complement fixation test is positive in 85% of patients and this test is believed to indicate the presence of live cysts. A precipitin test is positive in 65% of patients.

Liver biopsy

The histology of the liver is an indispensable aid to diagnosis. It is the only way of proving the presence of cirrhosis, and it may also establish the cause of this disease, as in haemochromatosis and hepatolenticular degeneration. It has proved invaluable in the assessment of chronic hepatitis and alcoholic liver disease.

PERCUTANEOUS LIVER BIOPSY

Since the liver is the largest organ in the body and is relatively constant in position, blind percutaneous biopsy is satisfactory in most patients.

Preparation

The nature of the investigation is explained to the patient; it is preferable to obtain written consent. Blood is taken for haemoglobin, prothrombin time and platelet count. If there is any reason to suspect these variables may change, then the tests should be repeated on the day of the biopsy.

A biopsy should not normally be performed unless the haemoglobin is over 10 g/100 ml, the platelet count over 100,000 mm^3 and prothrombin time no more than 3 sec longer than the control. Liver biopsy should also be avoided in the presence of substantial ascites or when extrahepatic cholestasis seems likely. In anxious patients premedication with diazepam by mouth may be helpful, but routine premedication is not necessary and may interfere with co-operation.

Procedure

The patient is positioned on the examination couch, or better still on the bed on which he will lie after the procedure. The patient lies supine close to the right edge of the bed. The right hand is placed behind the head which is supported by one pillow. The position of the liver is confirmed by percussion down the right side of the chest and abdomen. The puncture site is the point of maximal dullness between the anterior and mid-axillary lines. This usually lies in the 8th–10th intercostal spaces. The puncture site is positioned just above the appropriate rib, to avoid the vessels and nerves which run just below the ribs.

Occasionally, in case of difficulty or when a nodule can be palpated, a subcostal puncture may be made; this is a less satisfactory procedure even in the presence of marked liver enlargement.

It is not necessary to wear gowns or masks for this procedure, but the use of surgical gloves for the operator is recommended because of the potential risk of transmission of hepatitis. A paper sheet placed under the patient prevents any leakage of blood onto the bedding.

The patient is instructed to practise the breath-holding procedure: after a full aspiration and a full exhalation breath is held for a few seconds. During normal breathing the puncture site is thoroughly cleaned with alcohol swabs and infiltrated with 5 ml 2% lignocaine. The skin is anaesthetized with a fine needle, which is replaced by a 21 gauge needle to infiltrate down to the liver capsule with the breath held in expiration.

There are two types of needle in general use and both provide adequate biopsy samples. The Menghini suction biopsy needle has been longer established and requires a shorter period of penetration of the liver. The Tru-Cut sheathed biopsy needle is slightly more cumbersome to use and much more expensive.

The Vim-Silverman needle is obsolete as it distorts the sample.

Menghini needle (reusable)

The Menghini needle (Figure 27) is supplied in a variety of calibres and lengths. For routine use the 1.9 x 70 mm size is recommended. The slight theoretical advantage of smaller diameter needles is offset by the larger number of liver punctures required to obtain satisfactory tissue samples. The tip of the needle has a bevelled cutting edge. The needle is supplied with a blunt nail which fits inside the proximal shaft to prevent the sample being violently aspirated into the syringe, and with an external guard for the shaft to prevent too deep penetration of the liver; neither of these is essential. A trocar reminiscent of a sardine tin key is also supplied and is non-contributory.

The needle is attached to a 20 ml syringe containing 5 ml physiological saline. A skin incision is made with a small-blade scalpel and the needle is advanced through the chest wall to the pleura and diaphragm. Two millilitres of saline are injected to clear the needle. The patient then performs the breath-holding manoeuvre. Aspiration is applied to the syringe and the needle is rapidly introduced about 4 cm into the liver and then immediately withdrawn. Thereupon the patient is permitted to breathe normally. The needle is removed from the syringe, the nail removed and the core of liver tissue is gently extruded either onto filter paper first or directly into formol

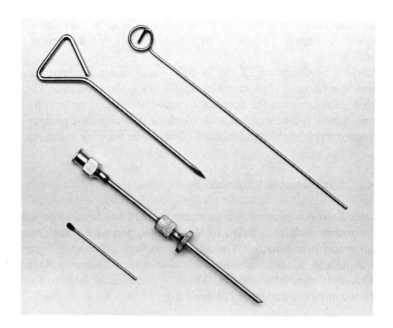

Figure 27(a) Menghini needle set displayed

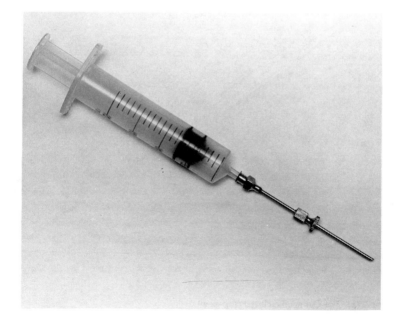

Figure 27(b) Menghini needle assembled (guard not in operating position)

saline, using the probe supplied. The contents of the syringe can be flushed through the needle into cytology fixative. If a satisfactory core (over 5 mm) is not obtained, then it is permitted to perform two more punctures at the same procedure.

Various modifications of the Menghini system are available. Disposable needles can be used. The Jamshidi needle is supplied with a locking syringe which does not require the operator to maintain traction on the plunger. The Surecut needle is also supplied with a locking syringe, to the plunger of which is attached a retractable trocar which obviates the need for saline injection.

Tru-Cut sheathed needle (disposable)

This needle requires more skill in operation, but has become popular partly because of its wide application to other biopsy procedures such as sampling prostate and breast tissue. The needle consists of an outer 2 mm cutting sheath through which is advanced a trocar with a 20 mm sampling groove positioned 10 mm from the tip. There is a choice of length of needle, of which the most convenient is 114 mm long.

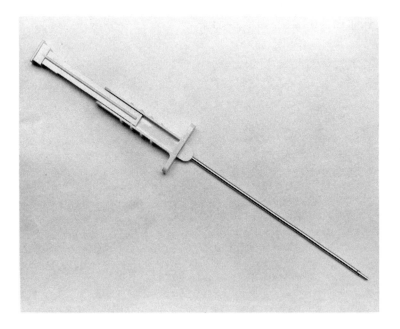

Figure 28(a) Tru-Cut needle closed (top view)

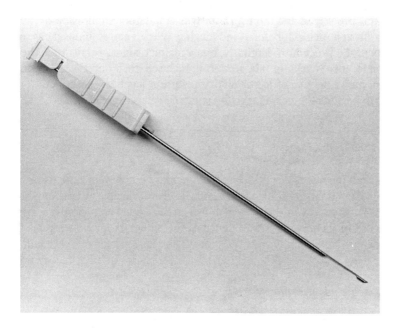

Figure 28(b) Tru-Cut needle open (side view)

After preparation, anaesthesia and skin incision with a scalpel, the needle is advanced to the liver capsule with the trocar retracted. The patient then holds the breath in expiration while the needle is advanced 4 cm into the liver with the trocar fully sheathed. The needle is then retracted to permit a sample of liver to bulge into the trocar sampling groove. The cutting sheath is then fully advanced holding the trocar steady, and the whole needle is removed.

Operators are recommended to practise the sequence of manoeuvres several times before puncturing patients and to consult the manufacturer's instruction leaflet supplied with each needle.

This procedure is an amendment of a previous one, designed to improve safety. Needles must never be reused.

Alternative techniques

Bleeding tendency

If the prothrombin time is prolonged, a course of vitamin K 10 mg i.v. or i.m.

daily for 3 days may cause it to return to normal. If the prothrombin time remains prolonged and the liver biopsy is mandatory an infusion of 2 units of fresh frozen plasma before and during percutaneous biopsy ensures the safety of the procedure. Similarly, if low platelet counts persist then the transfusion of two packs of platelets can be used to cover the procedure. In haemophilia the use of factor VIII transfusion has been described. It is possible to occlude the needle tract by injecting gelatin sponge.

Transvenous liver biopsy

This is an ingenious device, using transjugular hepatic vein catheterization for biopsy of patients with bleeding diathesis. The principle is that any haemorrhage is contained in the patient's own circulation. The procedure should be reserved for centres with experience of the catheterization technique. There is an appreciable failure rate and biopsy samples tend to be very small.

Peritoneoscopic liver biopsy

This is an alternative for the patient with a bleeding tendency, since direct haemostasis can be achieved. It allows targetted biopsy in non-homogenous liver disease and can be specially helpful in macronodular cirrhosis, lymphoma and metastatic disease. Naked-eye diagnosis should always be confirmed by histology.

Laparotomy

Liver biopsy at laparotomy is best done with biopsy needles to avoid spurious conclusions from the histology of the unrepresentative peripheral samples obtained with scissors or scalpel. Ideally the biopsy should be taken at the first procedure after opening the peritoneum. A laparotomy should never be performed for the *sole* purpose of obtaining a liver biopsy.

Young children

Percutaneous liver biopsy is feasible. Needles of 1.2 mm diameter are used. One assistant is required to talk to and gently restrain the patient if necessary. Another assistant immobilizes the liver by pressing on the left chest with the right hand, while pushing up the liver with the left hand. The procedure can mostly be performed with local anaesthesia, but a general anaesthetic may by required.

Ultrasonic guiding has been described, and if a lesion is identified, a *scintis-canning* needle biopsy can be targetted with a hand-held counter.

Aftercare

Gentle local pressure may be needed to stop oozing of blood. The biopsy wound is covered with an adhesive dressing. The patient is asked to lie as much as possible in the right lateral position for 4–6 hours. Pulse and blood pressure are recorded every 15 min for an hour, then hourly for 4–6 hours. The patient is warned to expect mild discomfort. If there is a severe pain at the biopsy site, in the epigastrum or right should tip, then an injection of pethidine 25–100 mg i.m. is given.

The procedure is mainly performed on in-patients, though it is increasingly used for *out-patients*; this is quite safe as long as patients can be observed for some hours after the procedure. Facilities must be available in order to admit those who develop important complications.

Complications

Serious morbidity occurs in about 5% of patients. The most important determining factor is the number of liver punctures. *Pain* is the commonest complication and is usually transient.

The major hazards are haemorrhage and bile leakage.

Bleeding into the pleura or peritoneum may require transfusion and open suturing. It is diagnosed by a rising pulse and falling blood pressure, without much pain. Bleeding is said to be more common from hepatoma. An intrahepatic haematoma is common and usually of no significance, though it may interfere with subsequent liver imaging techniques.

Bile leakage may occur from an intrahepatic gallbladder. It sometimes occurs from a large duct but this is uncommon if liver biopsy is avoided in extrahepatic cholestasis. Bile leakage usually causes pain and tachycardia; hypotension may also occur. Any serious bile leak requires early laparotomy, suturing of the liver and peritoneal toilet.

The mortality rate of liver biopsy is contentious, but probably lies between 1:3,000 and 1:10,000. The mortality rate depends on the type of patient undergoing biopsy and can be expected to be higher in patients with metastatic carcinoma.

Indications

(1)   Evaluation and monitoring of alcoholic liver disease.

189

(2)   Diagnosis of cirrhosis, chronic active hepatitis, drug jaundice, haemochromatosis, hepatolenticular degeneration, amyloid and sarcoid.

(3)   Diagnosis of hepatocellular carcinoma.

(4)   Diagnosis of metastatic carcinoma and lymphoma.

(5)   Diagnosis of hepatomegaly and splenomegaly.

(6)   Establishment of the cause of intrahepatic cholestasis.

(7)   Monitoring the progress of treatment in chronic active hepatitis and iron and copper storage diseases.

(8)   Confirmation of Dubin – Johnson syndrome (constitutional conjugated hyperbilirubinaemia).

(9)   Estimation of liver enzyme activity, e.g. glucuronyl transferase.

(10)   Occasionally in diagnosis of tuberculosis and pyrexia of unknown origin.

Contraindications to percutaneous biopsy

Absolute contraindications are an unco-operative patient, gross ascites, and suspected hydatid disease, haemangioma or peliosis hepatica.

Relative contraindications are proved extrahepatic cholestasis and a persistent bleeding tendency.

References

Perrault J, McGill DB, Ott BJ, Taylor WF. Liver biopsy: complications in 1,000 in-patients and out-patients. *Gastroenterology* 1978; **74**: 103 – 6

Greenwald R, Chiprut RO, Schiff ER. Percutaneous aspiration liver biopsy using a large-calibre disposable needle. *Am J Dig Dis* 1977; **22**: 1109 – 14

Menghini G. One-second needle biopsy of the liver. *Gastroenterology* 1958; **35**: 190 – 9

Bruguera M, Bordas JM, Mas P, Rodes J. A comparison of the accuracy of peritoneoscopy and liver biopsy in the diagnosis of cirrhosis. *Gut* 1974; **15**: 799 – 800

Trujillo NP. Peritoneoscopy and guided biopsy in the diagnosis of intra-abdominal disease. *Gastroenterology* 1976; **71**: 1083 – 5

Menghini G, Antonini R, Bruschelli P. Open abdomen liver biopsy by a modified one-second technique. *Am J Surg* 1977; **133**: 383 – 4

Rosch J, Lakin PC, Antonduic R, Dotter CT. Transjugular approach to liver biopsy and transhepatic cholangiography. *N Engl J Med* 1973; **289**: 227 – 31

Lebrec D, Goldfarb G, Degott C, Rueff B, Benhamou J-P. Transvenous liver biopsy. *Gastroenterology* 1982; **83**: 338 – 40

Riley SA, Ellis WR, Iriving HC, Lintott DJ, Axon AJR, Losowsky MS. Percutaneous liver biopsy with plugging of the needle tract. *Lancet* 1983; **2**: 436 – 7

Walker WA, Krivitt W, Sharp HL. Needle biopsy of the liver in infancy and childhood: a safe diagnostic aid in liver disease. *Paediatrics* 1967; **40**: 946 – 50

Rasmussen SN, Holm HH, Kristensen JK, Barlebo H. Ultrasonically-guided liver biopsy. *Br Med J* 1972; **2**: 500 – 2

Scheuer PJ. *Liver Biopsy Interpretation*. London: Balliere-Tindall 1988

Patrick RS, McGee JO'D. *Biopsy Pathology of the Liver*. London: Chapman and Hall 1988

Holund B, Poulsen H, Schlichting P. Reproducibility of liver biopsy diagnosis in relation to the size of the specimen. *Scand J Gastroenterol* 1980; **16**: 329 – 35

International Group. Alcoholic liver disease: morphological manifestations. *Lancet* 1981; **i**: 707–11

INTERPRETATION

Macroscopic appearance

It is often helpful to inspect the core of tissue which has been obtained. *Normal liver* is light brown or purple in colour. In *fatty liver* the biopsy is pale yellow. In *metastatic carcinoma* there may be white areas. In *Dubin–Johnson syndrome* the biopsy is black, while in the unconjugated hyperbilirubinaemia of the *Rotor syndrome* it is normal in colour.

In *cholestasis* dark bile plugs and heavy greenish-yellow pigmentation may be evident. In *cirrhosis* the liver appears non-homogenous and granular, with a gritty feel as the biopsy needle is inserted.

After rapid inspection the liver tissue should be immersed in formol saline for light microscopy. Other procedures necessitate the tissue samples being processed separately. For electron microscopy 4% iced glutaraldehyde is satisfactory. For cytology 95% alcohol or other special fixative is used. For liver enzyme assay fresh tissue should be transported on ice; it should be frozen rapidly if there is to be a delay in the analysis.

Histology

The value of the procedure depends on the adequacy of the size of the sample and the ability and experience of the pathologist. It is possible to diagnose acute viral hepatitis on a 5 mm core, but at least 15 mm is necessary for a reliable diagnosis of cirrhosis and chronic active hepatitis. Percutaneous and operative needle biopsies yield comparable results. Needle biopsies immediately after death are satisfactory, but autopsy histology is often difficult to interpret because of the frequency of centrilobular ischaemic necrosis. Surgical 'knife and fork' specimens yield large quantities of tissue, but a polymorphonuclear infiltrate and subcapsular fibrosis are very common even in apparently healthy livers.

Normal. The liver is arranged in regular units called acini. These are arranged around portal tracts, with a sinusoidal structure of mainly single cell plates between them and the central veins. In the portal tract are an arteriole, bile ducts, lymphatics and connective tissue. The wall of liver cells adjacent to the portal tract is known as the limiting plate. Between the parenchymal cells and the endothelial cells is the space of Disse containing tissue fluid and collagen and reticulin fibres. In the sinusoidal wall are the periodic acid-Schiff positive Kupffer reticuloendothelial cells, and also fat-storing lipocytes or Ito cells.

Some of the liver cells have double nuclei and some are polypoid, but mitotic figures are rare. Some nuclei contain glycogen. A few fat vacuoles occur in the cytoplasm, and there is little stainable iron. Near bile canaliculi brown granules of lipofuscin 'wear and tear' pigment are seen. With ageing, polyploidy becomes commoner, lipofuscin increases, and portal tract connective tissue becomes denser.

Acute viral hepatitis. There is extensive liver cell necrosis, worse around the centrilobular areas. It may be focal or confluent. Degenerate cells swell and become granular in appearance. There are rounded refractile eosinophilic bodies which reflect shrunken hepatocytes (Councilman bodies). A monocytic infiltration is observed especially round the portal tract. Marked centrilobular cholestasis may be evident. Orcein staining demonstrates the presence of the virus, which can also be shown by immuno-fluorescence. Liver biopsy is fairly reliable in diagnosis of viral hepatitis but does not distinguish it from drug hepatitis, so that an adequate history is important. It may be misleading if a biopsy is taken very early in the course of viral hepatitis.

Drug reactions. The histology in drug injury is variable and depends upon the nature of the drug. With some anabolic steroids there is centrilobular bile stasis; in chlorpromazine-type injury of the liver there is centrilobular bile stasis with variable portal inflammation, atypical proliferation of the bile ductules and many eosinophils; and in injury from monoamine oxidase inhibitors and halothane the histological picture is identical to that of viral hepatitis. An associated peripheral blood eosinophilia may give a clue to an idiosyncratic allergic drug reaction.

Cirrhosis. It is possible to obtain an apparently normal biopsy in cirrhosis which is macronodular, but as a general rule liver biopsy is a reliable method of proving the diagnosis.

The essential features are liver cell necrosis and nodular regeneration, with disorganization of the normal hepatic architecture. The 'activity' of the cirrhotic process, regardless of the aetiology, is assessed by the presence of 'piece-meal' necrosis, which produces an irregular border to the nodules, cellular infiltration and bile duct proliferation. In 'inactive' cirrhosis the nodules are smooth and well demarcated by relatively acellular fibrous bands.

Alcoholic liver disease. Abnormal liver histology is almost always associated with elevated gammaGT (and glutamate dehydrogenase) levels in the serum, but the histological lesion cannot be predicted from the clinical features. Some biopsy samples show normal architecture, though cytology of aspirated fluid usually shows necrotic liver cells, variable nuclear size and excess lymphocytes. The most common finding is increased *fat* in the parenchymal cells, which may be severe. *Fat granulomas* may occur. In *alcoholic hepatitis* there is extensive focal necrosis of liver cells with excess fat vacuoles (unlike viral hepatitis). *Mallory's hyaline bodies*, which stain deep reddish-purple with haematoxylin and eosin, are a helpful characteristic finding in both alcoholic hepatitis and cirrhosis, but they can occur in other conditions. Patients with alcoholic hepatitis may recover completely, die, or develop cirrhosis. The presence of perivenular sclerosis in alcoholic hepatitis may predict the development of cirrhosis. By contrast, megamitochondria carry a good prognosis. *Alcoholic cirrhosis* is not always distinguishable from other forms of cirrhosis, but the presence of Mallory's hyaline is an important clue. Some patients with alcoholic liver disease develop *chronic active hepatitis* and *hepatoma*.

Extrahepatic biliary obstruction. This may be difficult or impossible to differentiate by liver biopsy from causes of intrahepatic cholestasis. There are characteristically dilated and proliferating bile ducts with bile plugs.

Primary biliary cirrhosis. The histological appearance depends upon the stage of the disease. In the early stages histology is 'reasonably specific' with fibrosis and proliferation of the septal or interlobular bile ducts, local portal zone lymphocyte accumulations and peripheral cholestasis. At a later stage there is ductular destruction and encircling of the portal tracts by dense fibrous tissue. Eventually a form of cirrhosis ensues which is indistinguishable from cirrhosis of other types.

Chronic active hepatitis. Piece-meal necrosis of liver cells at the junction of connective tissue and parenchyma occurs, with extensive infiltrate of mononuclear cells (many of them plasma cells). Connective tissue increases and there is deposition of collagen to form new 'active' septa. The changes may be patchy throughout the liver.

Chronic persistent hepatitis. The main feature of inflammatory infiltration which is largely mononuclear and confined to the portal tract. Piece-meal necrosis and collagen deposition are absent.

Neonatal hepatitis. This shows many parenchymal giant cells, there is focal necrosis and intralobular ducts are identified. Although these features are absent in pure biliary atresia it is now considered that the conditions may represent extremes of a single disease spectrum.

Reduced or absent $alpha_1$-antitrypsin in the serum makes neonatal hepatitis more likely than atresia.

Malignant disease. In 75% of *metastatic disease* needle biopsies can demonstrate the tumour, but more than one biopsy may be necessary. In *hepatocellular carcinoma* a similarly high diagnostic rate may be achieved. If the lesion is diffuse, blind biopsy is adequate, but if it is a discrete tumour a targetted biopsy on the basis of a liver scan (ultrasonic or isotopic) yields better results.

Sometimes cytologic analysis of the washings from the Menghini needle shows malignant cells when the biopsy histology does not.

References

Desmet VJ, De Groote J. Histological diagnosis of viral hepatitis. *Clin Gastroenterol* 1974; **3**: 337–54

MacSween RNM. Pathology of viral hepatitis and its sequelae. *Clin Gastroenterol* 1980; **9**: 23–48

Cunningham D, Mills PR, Quigley, EMM *et al.* Hepatic granulomas: experiece over a 10 year period in the West of Scotland. *Q J Med* 1982; **51**: 162–70

Jimenez W, Pares A, Caballeria J *et al.* Measurement of fibrosis in needle liver biopsies: evaluation of a colorimetric method. *Hepatology* 1985; **5**: 815–8

Chedid A, Mendenhall CL, Tosch T *et al.* Significance of megamitochondria in alcoholic liver disease. *Gastroenterology* 1986; **90**: 1858–64

Abe H, Beninger PR, Ikejiri N, Setoyama H, Sata M, Tanikawa K. *Gastroenterology* 1982; **82**: 938–47

International Group. Alcoholic liver disease: morphological manifestations. *Lancet* 1981; **1**: 707–11

Dienes HP, Popper H, Arnold W, Lobeck H. Histologic observations in human hepatitis non-A, non-B. *Hepatology* 1982; **2**: 562–71

LIVER ASPIRATION

It is seldom that a diagnostic percutaneous liver aspiration without biopsy is undertaken. The main indication is the strong suspicion that an intrahepatic mass is an amoebic abscess. Hydatid cysts must not be aspirated by needle under local anaesthesia, although single pyogenic abscesses may be.

The technique is very similar to that for a liver biopsy. The procedure is relatively simple when the liver is enlarged and there is an abscess pointing in the subcostal region. The overlying skin and muscle is infiltrated with local anaesthetic and the patient is instructed to hold the breath in expiration. The needle which is attached to a 20 ml syringe is inserted into the mass or at the site of maximum liver tenderness. The needle is slowly withdrawn while gentle aspiration is performed until necrotic fluid material is obtained. The patient breathes shallowly while the abscess is aspirated. A short length of tubing connecting the needle to the syringe reduces the changes of damage to the liver capsule while the patient breathes.

It is also possible to perform a diagnostic aspiration through an intercostal space, but this is generally discouraged because of the danger of intrapleural soiling. The usual site for insertion of the needle is the 10th intercostal space and the liver is aspirated while the patient holds the breath. A short length of tubing connecting the needle with the syringe enables the patient to breathe quietly during the procedure.

The contents of an *amoebic abscess* are brown-red, 'anchovy sauce' necrotic material. Vegetative forms of *E. histolytica* are rarely found in the aspirated material and the final portion of the aspirate is more likely to contain the trophozoites. As amoebic pus usually coagulates after collection the pus is liquefied by the addition of one part hyaluronidase to five of pus. After incubation at 37°C for 1 hour, the samples are centrifuged at 1500 rpm for 5 min and the sediment examined for amoebae.

Modern imaging techniques permit accurate localization of an abscess and the precise insertion of the aspirating needle.

Liver imaging and manometry

The anatomy of the liver and spleen and the physiology of the portal circulation can be investigated in numerous ways. Some of the techniques are too specialized for general use, but many have found a place in routine diagnosis.

ULTRASONIC SCANNING

Ultrasound scanning (US) of the liver is a simple and reliable test for focal disease and for extrahepatic obstruction (Methods are briefly described in Chapter 9). Ideally a complete upper abdominal scan should be performed when liver scanning is requested, since valuable information about the gallbladder, bile ducts and pancreas may also be gained.

Interpretation

Liver metastases

Discrete echogenic areas and focal hypoechoic areas are the most common findings, but the patterns are extremely variable. Solid metastases over 2 cm in diameter and cystic ones larger than 1 cm are reliably detected. The right lobe of the liver lateral to the porta hepatitis is easiest to scan. Tumours up to 3–4 cm may be missed occasionally in other areas. The accuracy of ultrasonography in metastatic disease is about 80–90%, and it is probably as good or better than isotope scanning; but simple measurement of serum alkaline phosphatase has been reported to give similar results in known carcinomas, and this biochemical test may yet be the best method of screening for hepatic malignancy.

Hepatocellular carcinoma

This may be difficult to delineate. The ultrasonic consistency of the tumour may be similar to surrounding parenchyma, and the tumour may be diffuse with multiple small abnormal areas. A diagnostic success rate of around 60% is feasible with experience.

Cysts and abscesses

Ultrasonography is a very effective method of demonstrating hepatic cysts, and liver, subphrenic and other abdominal abscesses. Up to 100% accuracy in defining liver cysts and abscesses is possible and guided aspiration is readily performed if desired.

Jaundice

Ultrasonography is an extremely useful diagnostic tool in a patient with features suggestive of cholestatic jaundice.

Accurate ultrasonic visualization of the extrahepatic bile ducts is achieved in 93–97% of patients. The intrahepatic ducts are visualized only when dilated to a calibre of 4 mm or more. If extrahepatic ducts are of normal calibre they are seen in 60–80% of patients. Dilated extrahepatic ducts (<6–8 mm is the normal range, <10 mm if there has been a previous cholecystectomy) are regularly seen. In extrahepatic obstruction dilation of the extrahepatic ducts precedes dilation of the intrahepatic ducts. In intrahepatic cholestasis the bile ducts are usually normal, but there may be some dilation of intrahepatic (but not of extrahepatic) ducts.

There are some drawbacks to ultrasonography. Common duct stones, sclerosing cholangitis and ampullary strictures may escape detection; the distal common bile duct is obscured by bowel gas in some patients; enlargement of the pancreatic head may be due to either carcinoma or chronic pancreatitis; and gallstones may be incidental findings unrelated to the cause of jaundice.

Diffuse disease

High-amplitude echoes are found in *micronodular cirrhosis*, but also occur in fatty liver, hepatitis and congestive cardiac failure. This has been termed the 'bright liver'. The appearance is non-specific and insensitive, being often absent in macronodular cirrhosis, and ultrasonography is not recommended as a diagnostic procedure if these diseases are suspected. Portal hypertension and thrombosis of the portal and hepatic veins can also be detected.

Main indications

(1)   Diagnosis of cholestatic jaundice.
(2)   Diagnosis of cysts and abscesses.
(3)   Diagnosis of liver metastases.

References

Vicary FR, Shirley I. Ultrasound and hepatic metastases. *Br J Radiol* 1978; **51**: 596–8

Weaver RM, Goldstein HM, Green B, Perkins C. Gray scale ultrasonographic evaluation of hepatic cystic disease. *Am J Roentgenol* 1978; **130**: 849–52

Vallon AG, Lees WR, Cotton PB. Grey-scale ultrasonography in cholestatic jaundice. *Gut* 1979; **20**: 51–4

Joseph AEA, Dewsbury KC, McGuire PG. Ultrasound in the detection of chronic liver disease (the bright liver). *Br J Radiol* 1979; **52**: 148–88

Tudway D, Sangster G. Ultrasound diagnosis of portal vein thrombosis following splenectomy. *Postgrad Med J* 1986; **62**: 1153–6

Gupta S, Barter S, Phillips GWL, Gibson RN, Hodgson HJF. Comparison of ultrasonography computed tomography and ^{99}Tc liver scan in diagnosis of Budd-Chiari syndrome. *Gut* 1987; **28**: 242–7

Debongnie JC, Pauls C, Fievez M, Wibin E. Prospective evaluation of the diagnostic accuracy of liver ultrasonography. *Gut* 1981; **22**: 130–5

Hill MC, Dach JL, Shawker TH. Ultrasonography in portal hypertension. *Clin Gastroenterol* 1985; **14**: 83–104

Powell-Jackson P, Karani J, Ede R, Meire H, Williams R. Diagnosis of Budd-Chiari syndrome by liver ultrasound and colloid scintigraphy. *Gut* 1985; **26**: A568

Medhat A, Iber FL, Dunne M. A new quantitative u/s method for diagnosis of chronic parenchymal liver disease. *Gastroenterology* 1988; **94**: 157–62

Saverymuttu SH, Joseph AEA, Maxwell JD. Ultrasound scanning in the detection of hepatic fibrosis and steatosis. *Br Med J* 1986; **292**: 13–15

Taylor KJW. Liver imaging by ultrasonography. *Sem Liver Dis* 1982; **2**: 1–13

ISOTOPE SCANNING

In many departments isotopic liver scanning has been largely replaced by the more informative ultrasonic scanning as a rapid and simple technique for screening the liver. It remains useful in the assessment of cirrhosis with portal hypertension, diagnosis of large liver tumours and definition of liver and spleen size. The isotope most commonly used is the gamma-emitting [99m]technetium, which can either be administered as a colloidal sulphide or as labelled macroaggregates of albumin. The dose is 1 mcCi intravenously. The isotope is taken up by the Kupffer cells and has a half-life of 6 hours. [113m]Indium colloid is an equivalent alternative.

A supplementary procedure is to perform a second scan using either [67]gallium citrate, which is taken up in hepatocellular carcinoma and liver abscess, or [75]selenomethionine, which is taken up by tissues rapidly synthesizing protein such as hepatocellular carcinoma and the normal pancreas.

Clearance of ^{131}I-Rose Bengal, which is excreted by the hepatocytes, has also been used as a test of liver function. It has not established its place in adults, but has some use in the diagnosis of neonatal cholestatic jaundice.

Newer tests using iminodiacetic acid derivatives and [75]SeHCAT are under evaluation. These are certainly avidly and preferentially taken up by the liver.

Method

No special preparation of the patient is necessary and the patient need not be fasting. The patient is scanned in the supine position, and both anteroposterior and lateral scans are obtained. Scanning is commenced about 60 min after the intravenous injection of the isotope, when stabilization of the count rate indicates that maximal radioactivity has been reached over the liver. The scanning procedure takes between 1 and 2 hours depending upon the size of the liver. Recordings are made in black-and-white (the photoscan) and in colour (the scintiscan). Upon completion of the procedure the surface markings of the costal margins, xiphisternum and the liver, if enlarged, are marked on the scan to aid in its interpretation.

Interpretation

Normal liver. There is good, even uptake of the isotope with the maximum activity being registered over the right lobe. The spleen is clearly outlined with ^{99m}Tc.

Cirrhosis. A patchy appearance may be seen and when this is marked the liver may appear to have a number of filling defects. This has given rise to diagnostic difficulties with diffuse hepatic secondaries or even hypertension. Liver size may be either greatly reduced or increased.

Portal hypertension with collateral circulation. A characteristic pattern is seen: the small liver has a poor uptake, the large spleen avidly concentrates the ^{99m}Tc and there is clear outlining of the vertebral bodies.

Metastases. Areas of low activity are seen. Metastases of more than 3 cm are usually seen, but the technique has a low overall sensitivity of about 60%. Isotope scans do not differentiate between metastases, abscesses and cysts.

Hepatocellular carcinoma. This shows on the ^{99m}Tc scan as a filling defect, which may be rounded or extend as processes from the porta hepatis. A second scan with ^{75}selenomethionine or ^{67}gallium citrate shows the hepatocellular carcinoma as a 'hot' area and subtraction of the scans gives a positive result in 90% or more cases. *Hepatic abscesses* and *metastases* may show the same pattern, but the technique is not so reliable in these diseases and the ^{99m}Tc scan may be negative.

Indications

(1)   To define liver and spleen position and size.
(2)   Diagnosis of cirrhosis with portal hypertension.
(3)   Diagnosis of hepatocellular carcinoma.

References

Luthra MS, Scherl ND, Golden D, Collica CJ. Scintophotography in cirrhosis. *Arch Intern Med* 1968; **122**: 211–4
Lomas F, Dibos PE, Wagner HN. Increased specificity of liver scanning with the use of gallium citrate. *N Engl J Med* 1972; **286**: 1323–9

RADIOLOGY

There are a number of radiological techniques which are of value in the diagnosis of liver disease and its complications.

Plain abdominal radiograph

A film of the abdomen is of help in determining the liver and spleen size. An enlarged liver frequently causes diaphragmatic elevation though an enlarged spleen does not. Calcification in the liver substance is seen in benign tumours particularly haemangiomas, and in malignant tumours, abscesses and hydatid cysts. Less than 50% of hepatic hydatid cysts show calcification which may appear as a thin rim over part or all of the cyst surface, or the cyst may be extensively calcified in a reticular pattern. Air may be seen in the biliary tract and the identification of gallstones is of help in the icteric patient.

Barium studies

A barium swallow is of help in the identification of oesophageal varices, which are best demonstrated when the lower oesophagus is coated with a thin layer of barium. The oesophagus is slightly dilated and there are numerous filling defects which distort the vertical mucosal folds. The presence of varices indicates the opening of portasystemic anastomotic channels and is a sign of portal hypertension.

Varices are present when there is either intra- or extrahepatic obstruction to the portal circulation and do not necessarily indicate hepatic cirrhosis. They may be seen in the acute fatty liver, infectious and alcoholic hepatitis, and presinusoidal causes of portal hypertension such as schistosomiasis.

Percutaneous transhepatic cholangiography (PTC) (Figures 29, 30, 31)

This remains the definitive procedure for precise localization of the cause of extrahepatic obstruction before an abdominal operation is undertaken. Ultrasonography and computed tomography can often provide similar information.

Method

The patient is prepared as for a liver biopsy. It is important that a surgeon is informed when the procedure is to take place so that a laparotomy, if needed, can be performed without undue delay. Bile leakage and septicaemia may occur, even with the fine Chiba needle, and antibiotic cover starting immediately before the procedure is prudent. Gentamicin 80 mg and ampicillin 1 g for three doses at 8-hourly intervals is commonly used. Studies of blood haemostasis should be normal as for liver biopsy.

The patient is placed supine on the radiology table and the procedure is carried out under fluoroscopy. The needle is 15 cm long, 0.7 mm external diameter and fitted with a stylet (Figure 29). It is flexible so that the patient can breathe normally when it is in position.

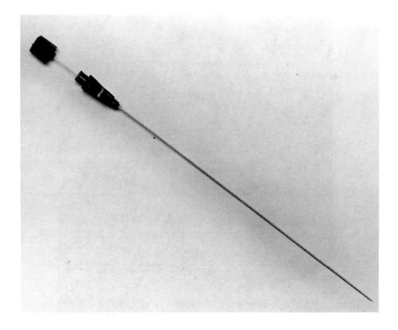

Figure 29 Chiba needle with stylet

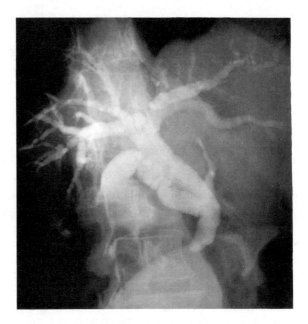

Figure 30 Percutaneous transhepatic cholangiogram showing a malignant stricture of the common bile duct (carcinoma of the pancreas)

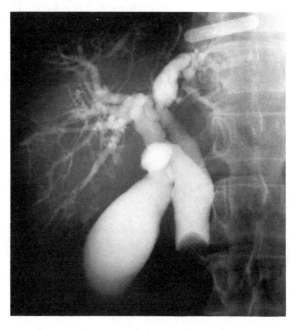

Figure 31 Percutaneous transhepatic cholangiogram showing a large gallstone impacted in the common bile duct

The skin is punctured in the 7th–8th right intercostal space in the mid-axillary line. The needle is advanced parallel to the table and is aimed two vertebral bodies below the junction of the diaphragm with the spine. After advancing fully the stylet is withdrawn. Because it may not be possible to aspirate bile even when the needle tip is positioned correctly, it is preferable to connect a syringe containing 50 ml 60% sodium meglumine diatrizoate via flexible tubing and inject a little contrast continuously as the needle is slowly withdrawn. Flow is centrifugal in bile ducts, as distinct from the centripetal flow of dye injected into portal veins, and the midline drainage in the hepatic veins. When a bile duct is entered contrast is injected and films are taken. If the needle is completely withdrawn without a bile duct being identified, five more attempts are permitted, using different puncture sites separated by 3–5 cm. Post procedure care is similar to that for a liver biopsy. If there is evidence of a bile leak immediate surgery is usually required.

Interpretation

The procedure identifies dilated ducts in 90–100% of cases, and has the added advantage of usually identifying the precise cause of obstruction. It also succeeds in demonstrating ducts in 65% of 'non-surgical' disorders. The technique is sufficiently accurate that if dilated ducts cannot be demonstrated, further evidence of extrahepatic obstruction in the jaundiced patient is required before undertaking a laparotomy. The overall mortality is 0.5% and morbidity is 5%. Fever occurs in 3.5% of cases, hypotension in 2%, bile leakage in 2.5% and bleeding in 1%.

In specialist centres PTC has an additional role, being used either for external biliary drainage or to insert a prosthesis in patients with malignant obstruction of the biliary tree, or to remove gallstones.

Transjugular cholangiography is feasible for the patient who has a bleeding tendency. Where PTC fails *minilaparotomy* or *laparoscopy* enables direct cholangiography before proceeding to full laparotomy.

Indications

(1)   Diagnosis of cholestasis.
(2)   Diagnosis of biliary strictures.
(3)   Diagnosis of hepatic duct carcinoma.

References

Okuda K, Tanikawa K, Emura T *et al.* Non-surgical percutaneous transhepatic cholangiography

– diagnostic significance in medical problems of the liver. *Am J Dig Dis* 1974; **19**: 21–36
Jain S, Long RG, Scott J, Dick R, Sherlock S. Percutaneous transhepatic cholangiography using the 'Chiba' needle – 80 cases. *Br J Radiol* 1977; **50**: 175–80

ENDOSCOPIC RETROGRADE CHOLANGIOPANCREATOGRAPHY (ERCP)

In general PTC is a better technique for demonstrating the biliary tree and ERCP is preferable for outlining the pancreatic duct system. ERCP can be used in the diagnosis of cholestasis where PTC is contraindicated, for example, coagulation defects, suspected hydatid disease or gross ascites. The success rate of cannulation and definition of dilated ducts is about 70–90%. There is a special hazard in extrahepatic obstruction in that a cholangitis rate of 20% may occur.

COMPUTED TOMOGRAPHY (Figures 32, 33)

This procedure provides good images of the liver and can demonstrate space-occupying lesions such as tumours, cysts and abscesses, as well as fatty liver. It is superior to isotope scanning and at least equivalent to ultrasonic scanning.

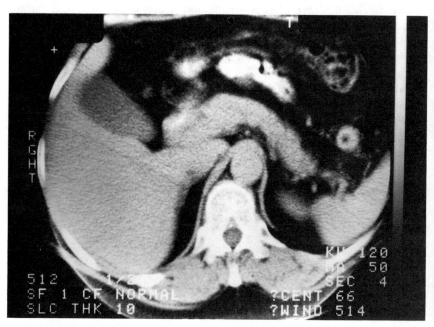

Figure 32 Normal CT scan showing liver, gallbladder, pancreas, aorta and crus of diaphragm

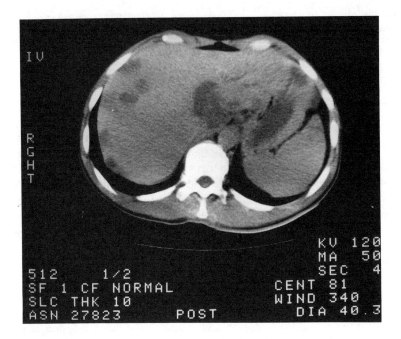

Figure 33 CT scan of the liver showing multiple low attenuation metastases from carcinoma of the stomach

Reference

Kreel L. Computerised tomography and the liver. *Clin Radiol* 1977; **28**: 511–81

NUCLEAR MAGNETIC RESONANCE IMAGING (MRI)

Though very expensive and not widely available as a result, MRI is superior to ultrasonography and isotope scanning in liver disease because of its greater specificity. It is probably also superior to computed tomography, and is likely to become more so with the development of technical advances and the use of contrast media such as gadolinium-DTPA and superparamagnetic ferrite–iron oxide particles.

References

Smith FW, Mallard JR, Reid A, Hutchinson JMS. Nuclear magnetic resonance tomography imaging in liver disease. *Lancet* 1981; **i**: 963–6

Smith FW, Mallard JR. NMR imaging in liver disease. *Br Med Bull* 1984; **40**: 194–6

Ferrucci JT. MR imaging of the liver. *Am J Roentgenol* 1986; **147**: 1103–16

Cherryman GR, Heron CW. Liver tumours: imaging techniques. *Clin Gastroenterol* 1987; **1**: 91–113

ARTERIOGRAPHY

Selective coeliac arteriography is of value in the investigation of patients with liver disease. The technique can be used to distinguish between benign lesions (such as hydatid cysts) and malignant tumours, which produce a characteristic distortion of the hepatic arterioles. The vasculature is also distorted in the cirrhotic liver. The technique can be used to outline the portal vein in patients who have undergone splenectomy or when splenic venography is contraindicated. The tip of the catheter is placed in the orifice of the superior mesenteric artery and contrast agent injected rapidly by hand while radiographic films are taken with a serial changer. The technique presents few problems for the radiological department versed in angiographic techniques.

Selective mesenteric arteriography has been used to define the collateral circulation in portal hypertension and to enable the direct infusion of pitressin to control haemorrhage. It is also used preoperatively to assist planning of surgery.

Diagnosis of cholestasis

There are many different causes of cholestasis, manifested by jaundice, itching, dark urine, conjugated hyperbilirubinaemia, and raised serum alkaline phosphatase. If the cause is extrahepatic, persistent and surgically remediable, it is important to proceed to surgery promptly to avoid secondary hepatocellular failure. By contrast, if the cause is intrahepatic then operation is contraindicated both because of the possibility of causing liver and renal failure and the absence of useful relieving surgical procedures.

The most common causes of extrahepatic obstruction are common bile duct gallstones and carcinoma of the head of the pancreas. The most common causes of intrahepatic cholestasis are alcoholic liver disease, drug toxicity, viral liver disease, and metastases. Rapid and safe diagnosis is essential if the correct management is to be employed. Sclerosing cholangitis and coexisting intrahepatic and extrahepatic causes for cholestasis may give rise to diagnostic problems.

At present the major techniques for the diagnosis of cholestasis are ultrasonic scanning, percutaneous transhepatic cholangiography, endoscopic retrograde cholangio-pancreatography, computed tomography and laparoscopy. The latter is the least useful. The chooice of technique to be used depends upon local expertise. In skilled hands equally accurate results can be obtained. A liver biopsy is not an appropriate *initial* procedure.

References

O'Connor KW, Snodgrass PJ, Swonder JE *et al.* A prospective study comparing four current non-invasive approaches in the differential diagnosis of medical versus surgical jaundice. *Gastroenterology* 1983; **84**; 1498–1504

Irving AD, Cushieri A. Laparoscopic assessment of the jaundiced patient. *Br J Surg* 1978; **65**: 678–80

PORTAL MANOMETRY AND SPLENOPORTOGRAPHY

Several ingenious procedures for measuring portal hypertension and performing portography (often undertaken simultaneously) have been devised. They are useful in the assessment of patients being evaluated for surgery, although it should be appreciated that the level of portal hypertension does not correlate in any way with the size of the oesophageal varices or the likelihood of their bleeding. Similarly, collateral vessels may be demonstrated at portography, but these may be perioesophagal rather than the submucosal veins which are prone to bleed.

Fibreoptic endoscopy and barium swallow examinations are the simplest and best methods of demonstrating the presence of oesophageal varices. Doppler probes are available for use at endoscopy to assess flow in varices.

References

MacCormack T, Martin T, Smallwood RH, Robinson P, Walton L, Johnson AG. Doppler ultrasound probe for assessment of blood-flow in oesophageal varices. *Lancet* 1983; **1**: 677–8

MANOMETRY

Splenic puncture

Method

The preparation of the patient and the precautions which are observed are similar to those for a liver biopsy.

The patient lies supine with the left arm behind the head. The upper limit of splenic dullness is defined while the breath is held in deep expiration. The site for insertion of the needle is selected midway between the mid and posterior axillary line and in that intercostal space below the upper level of splenic dullness. This is usually the eighth or ninth space.

The needle is advanced 2–3 cm into the spleen, the stylet is withdrawn and the patient is permitted to breathe gently. When the needle has been positioned correctly it is connected by means of a length of polyvinyl or polyethylene tubing which has been filled with normal saline to a pressure-recording transducer. The pressure is recorded while the patient breathes quietly. The zero level is taken at a point 5 cm below the sternal angle. Once the pressure measurements have been taken a splenic venogram may be performed. The tract may be occluded by injection of an absorbable gelatin sponge.

Interpretation

The normal intrasplenic pressure is less than 14 mmHg. Intrasplenic pressure is increased in cirrhosis to values between 17 and 35 mmHg, and similar values are found in extrahepatic portal vein obstruction.

Thus the intrasplenic pressure does not distinguish between intra- and extrahepatic causes of portal hypertension. An elevated intrasplenic pressure may be lowered and even fall within the normal range when there is a marked portasystemic collateral circulation or after bleeding from varices. The intrasplenic pressure relates closely to the pressure in the portal vein, which it usually exceeds by 2–4 mmHg.

Indications

(1) To confirm the presence of portal hypertension.
(2) To assess the success of a portacaval anastomosis. When there is a patent surgical shunt the intrasplenic pressure should return to normal values.
(3) Surgery for portal hypertension should be preceded by the measurement of portal pressure.

Reference

Brazzini A, Hunter DW, Darcy MD *et al.* Safe splenoportography. *Radiology* 1987; **162**: 607–9

Hepatic vein catheterization

This is a useful technique for the study of portal haemodynamics. It is not, however, essential to the management of a patient with liver disease and is not performed as a routine clinical investigation.

An open tip radio-opaque cardiac catheter is introduced under fluoroscopic control via an antecubital vein into the right or left lobe of the liver. The catheter is advanced until resistance is felt and no further progress is possible. This is the wedged position and pressures obtained in this position are believed to represent the portal vein pressure. The catheter is withdrawn so that it lies freely in the vein – the 'free' position. Hepatic vein pressures are recorded in the wedged and free positions.

The normal wedged hepatic vein pressure is between 6 and 12 mmHg and the free pressure is between 2 and 5 mmHg. The wedged hepatic vein pressure is increased when there is an intrahepatic cause for portal hypertension such as cirrhosis, but the pressure is normal when portal hypertension is due to presinusoidal or extrahepatic portal vein obstruction. The technique can be used to study portal pressures in the splenectomized subject and may be combined with radiological procedures to demonstrate the hepatic venous pattern.

It is possible to classify the causes of portal hypertension into pre- or postsinusoidal on the basis of the information provided by the intrasplenic and wedged hepatic vein pressure measurements (Table 4).

Table 4   Interpretation of portal manometry

Site of cause of portal hypertension	Intrasplenic pressure	Wedged hepatic vein pressure	Diagnosis
Presinusoidal	Elevated	Normal	Blocked portal or splenic vein; schistosomiasis; congenital hepatic fibrosis; myeloproliferative syndrome
Postsinusoidal	Elevated	Elevated	Cirrhosis; blocked hepatic veins; veno-occlusive disease

Intrahepatic pressure

The Chiba needle can be used to measure portal venous pressure. The procedure is as for PTC but an attempt is made to penetrate a portal vein which is identified by the centripetal flow of dye. Percutaneous manometry yields results similar to the wedged hepatic vein pressure (3–9 mmHg is normal, 14–45 mmHg in portal hypertension).

References

Ruzicka FF, Carillo FJ, D'Allessandro D, Rossi P. The hepatic wedge pressure and venogram versus the intra-parenchymal liver pressure and venogram. *Radiology* 1972; **102**: 253–8

Boyer TD, Triger DR, Horisawa M, Redeker AG, Reynolds TD. Direct transhepatic measurement of portal vein pressure using a thin needle. *Gastroenterology* 1977; **72**: 584–9

PORTOGRAPHY

This may be performed by direct puncture of spleen or liver, via the umbilical vein; or by selective splenic or superior mesenteric arteriography where the spleen is small or absent. Iodine contrast media and radioisotopes have both been used. Hepatic venography can be performed after wedged hepatic pressures have been taken.

Splenic venography (splenoportography)

This technique provides valuable information about the portal venous system. It is usually performed at the same time as the intrasplenic pressure is being measured. The radiological procedure should be combined with the measurement of intrasplenic pressure.

Method

The patient is prepared as for the measurement of the intrasplenic pressure. The patient is instructed to hold the breath in expiration and 40 ml of warm 45% sodium acetriozate ('Hypaque') is injected while a series of anteroposterior films are taken. The needle is immediately removed and the patient told to breathe gently.

The injection of the dye into the splenic pulp is usually painless. There is occasionally unpleasant flushing which rapidly subsides. Marked left shoulder-tip pain is felt when there is a sub-capsular spilling of the dye.

Interpretation

The early films are used to assess the portal collateral circulation and the later ones to assess the intrahepatic vascular pattern. The splenic and portal veins are identified and their calibre noted. The presence of collateral vessels is significant and gastric, oesophageal, splenic and lumbar venous channels may be seen. Filling may also occur of the inferior mesenteric, testicular or ovarian, and umbilical veins. Failure to visualize the portal vein suggests that it is blocked, but when there is a large collateral circulation the flow of the dye may be sufficiently deviated to prevent opacification of what is in fact a normal portal vein.

The intrahepatic venous pattern is seen as an initial 'vascular' phase when the rich branching portal vascular system is identified, and a later 'parenchymatous' phase when the liver shows as an intense homogenous shadow. In cirrhosis there is diminution and distortion of the intrahepatic radicles giving a sparse 'tree-in-winter' appearance. There is no filling of the intrahepatic radicles in extrahepatic obstruction to the portal vein. Tumours, cysts and abscesses cause distortion of the intrahepatic venous pattern.

Indications

(1)   To exclude extrahepatic causes of portal hypertension and to provide information about the portal vein in patients being considered for surgery for portal hypertension.
(2)   To diagnose the cause of an enlarged spleen.

Transumbilical portal venography

The place of this technique in demonstrating the portal venous system is still to be decided. Under local anaesthesia the umbilical vein is exposed at the umbilicus and hemissected. The collapsed lumen is teased open. The vein is patent in the majority of patients with cirrhosis. The vein is dilated until it admits a suitable catheter which is then advanced to the hepatic hilum. Care must be exercised on entering the left branch of the portal vein which can be damaged. An injection is made of the contrast material. There is excellent visualization of the interhepatic portal venous system, but the extrahepatic portal view is not always seen.

Transhepatic portography

The liver is punctured and the needle tip positioned in the portal vein near the hilum for manometry and then 20 ml contrast are injected. Ten radiographic films are taken at 1 second intervals.

Scintisplenoportography

Using splenic puncture, $5-8$ mCi ^{99m}Tc-labelled pertechnecate is injected and gamma-scanning undertaken, with counts and photography over the heart, right lobe of the liver and spleen. Three patterns of scintillation are defined:

(1) normal progress of isotope through splenic and portal vein and through the liver;
(2) abnormal collaterals but predominant flow to the liver;
(3) total diversion and no liver flow demonstrable.

An alternative technique includes the splenic injection of ^{99m}Tc-labelled albumin microspheres followed by ^{99m}Tc-labelled erythrocytes to define spleen and liver circulation. Percutaneous transhepatic portal vein catheterization with manometry, followed by injection of ^{99m}Tc-labelled albumin macroaggregates into the spleen and ^{131}I-labelled macroaggregates into the portal trunk, has also been used.

Hepatic venography

With a hepatic catheter in the wedged position, between 10 and 20 ml of warm 75% sodium acetriozate is injected rapidly by hand. A rapid succession of films is taken using a serial changer.

The normal liver demonstrates a delicate lattice network of fine venules. The larger hepatic veins are outlined as smooth regular branching vessels. In the cirrhotic liver the venule pattern is coarse and nodular, the larger hepatic veins are tortuous and irregular and there is a portal vein filling. Abnormal venous patterns are found in tumours and the Budd–Chiari syndrome.

References

Scott J, Long RG, Dick R. Percutaneous transhepatic obliteration of gastro-oesophageal varices. *Lancet* 1976; 2: 53–5

Smith-Laing G, Camillo ME, Dick R, Sherlock S. Percutaneous transhepatic portography in the assessment of portal hypertension. *Gastroenterology* 1980; 78: 197–205

Viamonte M, Peraras R, Russell E, Lepage J, Maer WL. Pitfalls in transhepatic portography. *Radiology* 1977; 124: 325–9

Hoevels J, Lunderquist A, Tyle NE. Percutaneous transhepatic portography. *Acta Radiol Diagn* 1978; 19: 643–55

Baron MG, Wolf BS. Splenoportography. *J Am Med Assoc* 1968; 206: 629–34

Kreel L. Radiology of the portal system. *Gut* 1970; 11: 620–6

Kashigawa T, Kamada T, Abe H. Dynamic studies of the portal dynamics by scintiphotography: The visualisation of portal venous system using ^{99m}Tc. *Gastroenterology* 1974; 67: 668–73

Syrota A, Vinot JM, Paraf A, Roucayrol J-C. Scintillation splenoportography: Haemodynamic and morphological study of the portal circulation. *Gastroenterology* 1976; **71**: 652–9

Okuda K, Suzuki K, Musha H, Arimizu N. Percutaneous transhepatic catheterisation of the portal vein for the study of portal haemodynamics and shunts. *Gastroenterology* 1977; **73**: 279–84

Viamonte M. Imaging techniques in portal hypertension. *Semin Liver Dis* 1982; **2**: 187–201

Gallbladder and bile ducts

Investigation of the biliary tree depends mainly on the demonstration of anatomical changes by radiology, or ultrasonic and isotope scanning techniques. Serum biochemistry may lend support to diagnosis, but is usually non-specific. Studies of biliary physiology have not found their way into routine clinical practice. Duodenal drainage with examination of bile-rich fluid is seldom used in making a diagnosis of gallbladder disease, though in gallstone disease cholesterol crystals indicate cholesterol-rich stones, and microspheroliths indicate mineral/pigment stones.

RADIOLOGY

Plain abdominal radiograph

Ten to twenty percent of gallstones are sufficiently calcified to be visible on the upper right side of the abdomen. Sometimes the calcification is homogenous, but often it shows an internal laminar pattern which is helpful in diagnosis. Gallstones may either have rounded contours, or straight edges if they have been pressed against other stones. Multiple small irregular calcified stones are frequently composed of calcium bilirubinate. Pure cholesterol stones are radiolucent.

Occasionally larger gallstones show internal fractures with hyperlucent lines radiating from the centre. This is called the tri-fin or Mercedes–Benz sign and can be detected even in the absence of calcification. The position of gallstones usually requires confirmation by supplementary procedures. Calcium deposits are occasionally seen in the gallbladder wall: the 'porcelain gallbladder'. Even less often bile contains a large amount of calcium salts in suspension: 'limy' or 'milk of calcium' bile, which outlines the biliary tree.

Gas in the biliary tree occurs in infections with gas-forming organisms is called emphysematous cholecystitis. It also occurs when there is a fistula between the intestine and gallbladder or bile ducts and after some operations to the biliary tree. Gas can also occur when there is an incompetent sphincter of Oddi, which may result from sphincteroplasty.

Oral cholecystography (Figures 34, 35)

This remains a popular method of demonstrating gallstones in a functioning gallbladder. It is, however, superseded by ultrasonography in most centres. Oral cholecystography is less useful in acute cholecystitis when cystic duct obstruction occurs. Good results are obtained by experienced radiographers and the technique is economical of radiologists' time.

Method

A plain radiograph of the abdomen is taken prior to ingesting the contrast medium. An opaque medium is administered orally, and this is absorbed from the intestinal tract, excreted by the liver, concentrated in the gallbladder and discharged via the bile ducts into the intestine. A variety of tri-iodo organic iodine compounds may be used for this purpose and a popular agent is iopanic acid 3 g. This is taken as 6 x 500 mg tablets with a normal evening meal on the evening before the examination. Thereafter the patient is asked to fast until the radiographic examination the following day.

An alternative technique is to use 6 g iopanic acid spread out over $1-2$ days prior to the examination. This may yield a higher proportion of positive results at the first examination.

Some departments routinely use a laxative with the preparation. As this may interfere with the absorption of the contrast medium, and as intestinal gas causes much more difficulty with interpretation than faeces, it cannot be recommended.

Radiographic films of the full gallbladder are obtained between 12 and 16 hours after the ingestion of the opaque medium, including films in both erect and horizontal postures. In cases of poor opacification tomography is helpful.

Gallbladder contraction is then stimulated by either a physiological stimulus such as eating two eggs, a cheese roll or a bar of chocolate, or by slow intravenous injection of cholecystokinin (CCK) 33 units. Larger doses of cholecystokinin and proprietary emulsions cannot be recommended as they are very prone to causing abdominal distress and vomiting. Caerulin is an alternative pharmaceutical preparation but has no definite practical advantages. Further radiographic films are taken after gallbladder contraction, which occurs $30-60$ min after an oral stimuli and $10-20$ min after intravenous CCK.

Contraction films may show calculi which were not visible in the filled gallbladder, and it is at this stage that it may be possible to visualize the cystic duct. The common bile duct is only occasionally delineated clearly by oral cholecystography. Failure of gallbladder function on cholecystography is not certain evidence for disease, and it is advisable to repeat the examination at least once. This may conveniently be done after an initial series of films

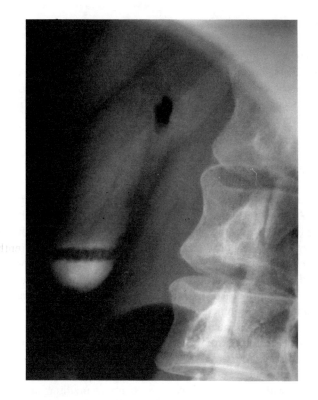

Figure 34 Oral cholecystogram showing floating gallstones

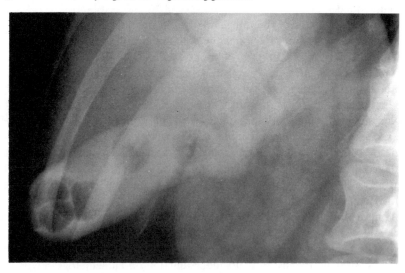

Figure 35 Oral cholecystogram showing radiolucent gallbladder stones, two with internal fractures (Mercedes – Benz sign)

following a 3 g dose of iopanic acid by giving a further dose of 3 g iopanic acid on the day of the unsatisfactory examination and repeating the films the next day. Alternatively, some other test such as ultrasonography or infusion cholangiography should be undertaken.

Interpretation

There are two definite oral cholecystogram appearances which demonstrate unequivocal evidence of organic gallbladder disease. One is when there are gallbladder stones, and the other is the presence of contrast in the bile ducts but no gallbladder filling.

In 5% of examinations there is evidence of some abnormality of the gall-bladder wall such as cholesterolosis, adenomyomatosis, papillomas, prominent spiral valves and a Phrygian cap. These occur independently of gall-stones and cholecystitis, and are not proof of symptomatic biliary disease.

Cholesterolosis of the gallbladder is suspected when there is an uneven mucosal contour with single or multiple filling defects. Adenomyomatosis of the gallbladder may show as a solitary filling defect, as a segmental stricture which must be distinguished from a 'Phrygian cap' (in which the septum is thinner and the distal segment contracts proportionately with the proximal segment), and as a diffuse condition which can be recognized by the contrast-filled Rokitansky–Aschoff sinuses. In cancer of the gallbladder there is usually no function of the gallbladder, which generally contains gallstones.

A meticulous radiological technique is required for oral cholecystography and, given this it is one of the most accurate of radiological investigations. The method can detect abnormality with a 95–99% accuracy. It gives positive evidence of 70% and presumptive evidence of 98–99% of gallstones, and probably detects 95% of significant cholecystitis.

Failure to outline the gallbladder also occurs if there is impaired absorption of the contrast medium. This may result from vomiting, delayed gastric emptying and diarrhoea. In such circumstances no conclusions can be drawn regarding gallbladder function. Oral cholecystography is not undertaken when there is liver cell dysfunction, because no satisfactory excretion of the dye is obtained when the serum conjugated bilirubin concentration is greater than 50 mcmol/l. Difficulty may also occur in anicteric patients with cholestasis. In the absence of parenchymal liver disease or hypermotility of the gut the failure to visualize the gallbladder after two attempts at cholecystography (the second being with a double dose of the contrast agent) may be accepted as evidence that the organ is diseased. The technique should be avoided in renal failure, where it is often ineffective and also hazardous.

A problem which is sometimes encountered is the patient with classical biliary colic or acute relapsing pancreatitis in whom the oral cholecystogram is normal. In some of these cases ultrasonography (or repeat cholecystography) reveals stones. In cholecystitis without demonstration of gallstones on cholecystography, hyperlucent fat in the gallbladder wall may provide a clue to the diagnosis in about 50% of cases.

References

Berk RN, Loeb PM, Goldberger LE, Sokolof FJ. Oral cholecystography with iopanic acid. *N Engl J Med* 1974; **290**: 204–10

Levesque HP. Sabulography. *Am J Roentgenol* 1970; **110**: 214–25

Burhenne HJ, Obata WG. Single-visit oral cholecystography. *N Engl J Med* 1975; **292**: 627–8

Melnick GS, Locurcio SB. The 'nonvisualised' gallbladder. A tomographic re-evaluation. *Diagn Radiol* 1973; **108**: 513–5

Mujahed Z, Evans JA, Whalen JP. The non-opacified gallbladder on oral cholecystography. *Radiology* 1974; **112**: 1–3

Andersson A, Bergdahl L. Disease of the gallbladder in patients with normal cholecystograms. *Am J Surg* 1976; **132**: 322–4

Russell JGB, Keddie NC, Gough AL, Galland RB. Radiology of acalculous gallbladder disease – a new sign. *Br J Radiol* 1976; **49**: 420–4

ULTRASONOGRAPHY (Figure 36)

Static grey-scale ultrasonography is an accurate method for diagnosis of gallbladder stones, and the overall detection rate is 85–96%. High-definition real-time ultrasonic scanning is very rapid and simpler to perform, and yields a 96% accuracy without missing any stones visible on conventional oral cholecystography.

Gallstones over 3 mm in size can be detected as mobile structures within the gallbladder, whose wall is often thickened. Those stones over 5 mm in diameter produce prominent acoustic shadows which assist interpretation. The presence of calcium in stones increases the ultrasonic definition.

The thickness of the gallbladder wall may be a clue to disease. It is ⩾2 mm in 97% of asymptomatic subjects without gallstones and ⩽3 mm in 45% with gallstone disease. Large carcinomas of the gallbladder are readily seen, as are mucoceles.

Failure to obtain an image of the gallbladder is uncommon, but may also be a sign of disease.

Ultrasonography is useful for measuring bile duct calibre but is not as accurate as the infusion cholangiogram for detecting duct stones. It readily defines choledochal cysts in children. Ultrasonography can be employed at laparotomy using a transducer held adjacent to bile ducts and pancreas. This could replace the operative cholangiogram.

Ultrasonic gallbladder scanning is very useful for evaluation of the nonfunctioning gallbladder or after a failed cholecystogram. High-definition

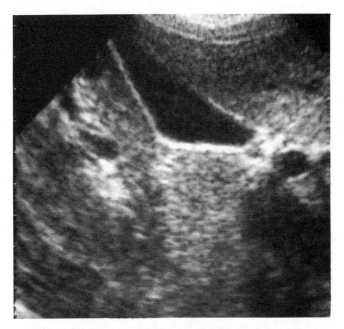

Figure 36(a) Abdominal ultrasound showing normal gallbladder

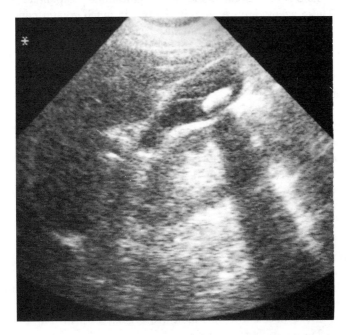

Figure 35(b) Abdominal ultrasound showing gallstone as an echogenic focus with acoustic shadowing

real-time scanning largely replaces the oral cholecystogram. Real-time scanning is being used to study gallbladder motility and may well prove to be of value in the definition and diagnosis of 'biliary dyskinesia'.

References

Cooperberg PL, Burhenne HJ. Real-time ultrasonography: diagnostic technique of choice in calculous gallbladder disease. *N Engl J Med* 1980; **302**: 1277–9

Anderson JC, Harned RK. Grey-scale ultrasonography of the gallbladder. *Am J Roentgenol* 1977; **129**: 957–77

Finberg HJ, Birnholz JC. Ultrasound evaluation of the gallbladder wall. *Radiology* 1979; **133**: 693–8

Yeh HC. Ultrasonography and computed tomography of carcinoma of the gallbladder. *Radiology* 1979; **133**: 167–73

Lane RJ, Glazer G. Intraoperative B-mode ultrasound scanning of the extrahepatic biliary system and pancreas. *Lancet* 1980; **2**: 334–7

Mirvis SE, Vainwright JR, Nelson AW *et al.* The diagnosis of acute acalculous cholecystitis. *Am J Roentgenol* 1986; **147**: 1171–5

IODINE CHOLANGIOGRAPHY

Organic iodine compounds may be administered intravenously and popular agents include sodium iodipamide, methylglucamine iodipamide and ioglycamide. These agents are excreted in the bile in much greater concentrations than the oral cholecystographic media. Their visualization does not depend upon the continuing ability of the gallbladder mucosa.

Method

Patients with a serum bilirubin less than 50 mcmol/l, who are not iodine-sensitive, and who are not in renal failure are suitable for the test.

An infusion of 4 mg/kg ioglycamide is given over 1 hour and films including tomograms are taken from 10–60 min after the infusion has commenced. This method avoids the flushing, nausea and vomiting which may be associated with bolus dose intravenous injection of contrast.

Interpretation

Bile duct calibre increases with age and after cholecystectomy. However, the normal common bile duct in adults is always less than 10 mm in diameter. Dilation of the duct above this indicates organic obstruction, where values from 12–25 mm are commonly seen.

The technique detects calculi and strictures. It may define anomalous bile ducts, retained cystic ducts and bile duct carcinomas. It is less accurate than operative cholangiography. Visualization of the ducts but not the gallbladder in a patient who has not had a cholecystectomy indicates organic disease. This may be either acute cholecystitis, or a stone impacted in the cystic duct or a chronically inflamed non-functioning gallbladder. Intravenous agents should not be used for the sole purpose of outlining the gallbladder which is best demonstrated by oral contrast media. Renal failure is a relative contraindication and alternative procedures should be considered. Some authorities no longer consider this procedure valid, but it still has a place as a reserve investigation.

References

Bell GD, Frank J, Fayadh M, Smith PLC, Fry IK. Ioglycamide (Biligram) studies in man. *Br J Radiol* 1978; **51**: 191–5

Goodman MW, Ansell HJ, Vennes JA, Lasser RB, Silvis SE. Is intravenous cholangiography still useful? *Gastroenterology* 1980; **79**: 642–5

INFUSION TOMOGRAPHY

This is a useful method in the diagnosis of acute cholecystitis, and where it is preferable to conventional infusion cholangiography. One hundred and fifty millilitres of 60% meglumine ditriazoate is mixed with 150 ml 5% dextrose and given by rapid intravenous infusion.

Linear tomograms of the anterior third of the upper right abdomen are taken. A positive result is an opacified ring caused by uptake of contrast by polymorphs in the inflamed gallbladder wall.

The test is accurate in 95% of cases.

Reference

Moncada R, Cardooso M, Danley R, Rodriguez J, Kimura K, Pickleman J, Brandly J. Acute cholecystitis: 137 cases diagnosed by infusion tomography of the gallbladder. *Am J Roentgenol* 1977; **129**: 583–5

ULTRASONOGRAPHY IN BILE DUCT DISEASE

This is a useful method of determining bile duct calibre, which increases slightly with age, but much more so in choledocholithiasis and in obstructive jaundice.

The role of ultrasound in locating bile duct stones is more problematical.

Initial experience was very disappointing, but improved techniques especially when combined with assessment of symptoms and serum biochemistry give reliable results.

The use of ceruletide may further enhance results.

References

Wermke W, Schulz H-J. Sonographic diagnosis of bile duct calculi: prospective study in 222 cases with choledocholithiasis. *Ultraschall* 1987; **8**: 116–20

Okuda K, Tsuchiya Y. Ultrasonic anatomy of the biliary system. *Clin Gastroenterol* 1983; **12**: 49–64

Mendelson RM, Tobin MV, Gilmore IT. Bile duct measurements after ceruletide as an aid to the ultrasound diagnosis of choledocholithiasis. *Gastrointest Radiol* 1988; **13**: 41–4

Kaude JV. The width of the common bile duct in relation to age and stone disease. *Eur J Radiol* 1983; **3**: 115–7

Tobin MV, Mendelson RM, Lamb GH, Gilmore IT. Ultrasound diagnosis of bile duct calculi. *Br Med J* 1986; **293**: 16–7

COMPUTED TOMOGRAPHY

This gives good results in gallstone disease, gallbladder cancer and obstructive jaundice, but other cheaper techniques do so too and should normally be the first choice.

A special use is in the evaluation of stones for non-surgical therapy. Radiolucent stones may have significant calcification precluding a successful dissolution therapy, and this is indicated by CT density greater than 90 Hounsfield units. Since this type of treatment can be very prolonged it is helpful to use CT as a screen to exclude some of the cases where failure can be predicted.

It seems likely that MRI will eventually reach the stage where it is possible to make exact chemical analyses of stones within the patient.

ISOTOPE SCANNING

[99m]Technetium compounds have been developed which are rapidly excreted by the liver even in the presence of cholestatic obstructive jaundice. Two which have been well evaluated are ^{99m}Tc-labelled dimethyl-acetanilide iminodiacetic acid (^{99m}Tc-HIDA) and ^{99m}Tc-labelled pyridoxylidene glutamate (^{99m}Tc-PG). The procedure is used for the diagnosis of acute cholecystitis and is helpful in the differential diagnosis of acute abdominal pain. Scans should be performed within 48 hours of admission to hospital.

Method

The patient is fasted for 4 hours. Two millicuries of ^{99m}Tc-PG is normally injected intravenously, but 5 mCi is used if the patient is icteric. Five to ten millicuries of ^{99m}Tc-HIDA is an alternative. The patient is then scanned by gamma-camera with dynamic studies and serial photographs every 10 min for 1 hour. If no gallbladder image is seen then the scan is repeated at 3–4 hours. If desired the nature of a gallbladder image may be confirmed by scanning 10–20 min after intravenous CCK 33 units.

Interpretation

A positive scan (no gallbladder activity) is always seen in acute cholecystitis, and in about half the patients with other gallbladder diseases. A negative scan (gallbladder activity) excludes acute cholecystitis but does not necessarily mean the gallbladder is normal. In infancy failure of excretion after liver uptake indicates biliary atresia.

This technique has a particular role in the diagnosis of persistent cholestatic jaundice in the early months of life. Some 60% of such patients have biliary atresia which may require surgery, but 25% have neonatal hepatitis of one form or another and this is a contraindication to operative intervention.

^{131}I-Rose Bengal

This is obsolete for adults, but still used in infantile jaundice.

Method

The patient is given Lugol's iodine three drops daily for 3 days to block the thyroid uptake of free radioiodine. ^{131}I-labelled Rose Bengal 1 mcCi/kg is given intravenously. Stools are collected for 72 hours and the amount of radioactivity is expressed as a proportion of the administered dose.

Interpretation

A normal result is excretion of less than 10% of the administered dose in 3 days, and this occurs in 93% with biliary atresia and only 28% with neonatal hepatitis. This method is therefore important in the evaluation of neonatal jaundice.

References

Weissman HS, Frank MS, Bernstein LH, Freeman LM. Rapid and accurate diagnosis of acute cholangitis with ^{99m}Tc HIDA cholescintigraphy. *Am J Roentgenol* 1979; **132**: 523–8

Weissman HS, Frank M, Rosenblatt R, Goldman M, Freeman LM. Cholescintigraphy, ultrasonography and computerised tomography in the evaluation of biliary tract disorders. *Semin Nucl Med* 1979; **9**: 27–35

Mowat AP, Psacharopoulos HT, Williams R. Extrahepatic biliary atresia versus neonatal hepatitis. *Arch Dis Child* 1976; **51**: 763–70

Laws JW. Non-invasive radiology. *Clin Gastroenterol* 1984; **13**: 1–286

Lecklitner ML, Austin AR, Benedetto AR, Growcock GW. Positive predictive value of choles-cintigraphy in common bile duct obstruction. *J Nucl Med* 1986; **27**: 1403–6

Cabellon S, Brown JM, Cavanaugh DG. Accuracy of the hepatobiliary scan in acute cholecystitis. *Am J Surg* 1984; **148**: 607–8

OTHER TECHNIQUES

Barium radiology

Barium meals and hypotonic duodenography can demonstrate ampullary carcinomas. Stones impacted in the terminal common bile duct cause duodenal oedema with a smooth indentation into the inner duodenal loop.

Operative and postoperative cholangiography

At the time of cholecystectomy the cystic duct is cannulated and iodine contrast such as diatrizoate is injected. Good images of the common duct and both hepatic ducts are obtained. This procedure eliminates the risk of unsuspected retained stones, known to occur in up to 4% of patients who are followed after cholecystectomy. It also detects the rarer hepatic and bile duct carcinomas. At present the consensus view is that operative cholangiography should be undertaken on all patients undergoing cholecystectomy for gallstones unless there has been careful preoperative screening with either PTC or ERCP.

Both flexible and rigid choledochoscopes (cholangioscopes) are available for the same purpose; these usually require the common duct to be opened for their insertion and do not offer entirely satisfactory views of the distal common bile duct.

Where duct stones have been removed it is usual to leave a T-tube in place and to confirm clearing of calculi by repeating the cholangiogram through the tube immediately before it is removed.

Endoscopic retrograde cholangiography is useful where other methods fail to demonstrate bile duct stones, and is claimed to give an overall accuracy of 92%. This technique can also be used to fill the gallbladder and intrahepatic ducts.

Biliary physiology

Manometry of the biliary tract using catheters passed at ERCP, percutaneous transhepatic puncture, T-tubes and direct intraoperative puncture can be performed. It is possible to test the response of the pressure recording to cholecystokinin, anticholinergics, spasmolytics and opiates.

The interpretation of these findings is difficult, though some authorities have taken high pressures to indicate a disease which has been termed 'biliary dyskinesia'.

Gallbladder emptying can conveniently be studied by planimetry of serial oral cholecystogram films, by gamma-scanning after intravenous ^{99m}Tc-HIDA, or by real-time ultrasonography. Emptying can be provoked by infusions of CCK or dietary fat. It is more rapid in men, in the elderly, and at the midpoint of the menstrual cycle. In gallstone disease many gallbladders do not function at all, but in the remainder emptying is said to be unduly rapid. There is a wide overlap with normal values.

Cholecystokinin. The availability of this hormone and its analogues has led to the introduction of tests based on the reproduction of symptoms suspected of a biliary origin, demonstration of biliary motility patterns and analysis of bile-rich duodenal fluid. None is reliable in diagnosis.

Bacteriology

Anaerobic and aerobic cultures of bile aspirated at operation show that organisms are present in 30–56% of gallbladders in patients with biliary disease and in 20% of controls. Common duct bile is infected in 75% of patients with choledocholithiasis. There is no relationship between the profusion of bacterial isolates and biliary symptoms, though knowledge of organisms may guide antibacterial therapy.

Reference

Dye M, MacDonald A, Smith G. The bacterial flora of the biliary tract and liver in man. *Br J Surg* 1978; **65**: 285–7

Ascites and the peritoneum

The aetiology of ascites may be obvious from the history and physical examination. However, it is generally necessary to examine the fluid microscopically, chemically and bacteriologically because even when the cause is clinically apparent, for example hepatic cirrhosis and portal hypertension, it may not be possible to exclude either superimposed infection or hepatocellular cancer.

ABDOMINAL PARACENTESIS

Diagnostic paracentesis is a simple technique and can easily be undertaken in all patients presenting for the first time with ascites unless there is a specific contraindication.

Method

The usual site for aspiration is in the right or left lower quadrant midway between the umbilicus and the anterior superior iliac spine. A 21 gauge needle may be used to inject the local anaesthetic and a similar size needle can then be inserted through the peritoneum for the paracentesis. Other suitable needles are those used for lumbar and cisternal puncture. When there is a very tense ascites it is often possible to insert a fine needle without using local anaesthetic. After a sufficient volume of fluid has been withdrawn for examination the needle is removed and a gauze dressing is applied to the wound.

Complications

These are rare. Occasionally an abdominal wall vein is penetrated. The procedure may be followed by a leak of fluid from the injection site when the ascites is very tense. A skin suture inserted after aspiration may prevent this, but not infrequently the leak only stops when the ascites has been relieved.

Interpretation

Appearance

Ascitic fluid which is a *transudate* is clear and straw-coloured. An *exudate* may also be clear but the fluid is usually cloudy and opalescent becaues of a high cell content. Trauma, malignant disease or tuberculous disease of the peritoneum may cause the fluid to be bloodstained. The fluid has a high mucoid content when pseudomucinous tumours have invaded the peritoneum.

Microscopic examination

Five millilitres of the ascitic fluid are added to a tube containing anti-coagulant, centrifuged for 10 min and a smear made of the deposit. A rough estimate is made of the number of cells and a differential count is undertaken. The presence of many polymorphonuclear leucocytes suggests non-tuberculous infection while a high lymphocyte count suggests tuberculosis or lymphoma. The unstained smear may be examined for microfilaria and trypanosomes, or it can be fixed and stained with either Leishman or Giemsa stain.

The spun deposit may be stained and examined for malignant cells by a trained cytopathologist. An accuracy of about 86% correct positive diagnosis is achieved. There is much difficulty in identifying cells when there has been ascites of long duration such as with cirrhosis of the liver. Exfoliated mesothelial cells are a particular cause of confusion and can be mistaken for malignant cells.

A counting chamber can be used for cell counts but caution must be exercised in the interpretation of the result when there is contamination with red blood cells.

In *transudates*, for example alcoholic liver disease, the mean cell count is $280 \pm 370/mm^3$.

In *exudates* the count is usually over $500/mm^3$. Exudates associated with carcinoma have an average cell count of $690/mm^3$ (with mixed cellularity); tuberculous exudates characteristically many lymphocytes (92%). Two conditions with very high counts, averaging $7000/mm^3$, are lymphomas where nearly 70% of cells are lymphocytes, and spontaneous bacterial peritonitis in which the cells are almost entirely polymorphs.

Chemical analysis

A *protein content* of less than 25 g/l suggests that the fluid is a transudate.

This is usually the case in heart failure, cirrhosis of the liver, nephrosis and other conditions associated with severe hypoproteinaemia. A protein concentration greater than 25 g/l suggests the presence of an exudate. This is found in acute peritoneal infections, tuberculous peritonitis and metastatic malignant disease involving the peritoneum; but occasionally a high protein content is encountered in cirrhosis in the absence of infection or malignant disease. The ascitic fluid may contain a high protein content in patients with myxoedema and endomyocardial fibrosis.

The *amylase* concentration of the ascitic fluid may be increased in patients with acute pancreatitis and pancreatic pseudocyst. Occasionally a perforated peptic ulcer will be associated with amylase-rich ascitic fluid.

Bacteriological examination

At least 10–20 ml of the ascitic fluid is sent for culture. When tuberculosis is suspected a large volume of the fluid is sent to the laboratory in a bottle containing sodium citrate to prevent the fluid from clotting. The tubercle bacilli may be sought by smear, culture or guinea-pig innoculation, but the diagnosis of tuberculous peritonitis is established by bacteriological methods in only 50% of patients.

Diagnostic paracentesis in the acute abdomen

The technique is a modification of that used when there is ascites. A 21-gauge needle is inserted under local anaesthesia into the peritoneal cavity at four sites: the right and left upper and lower quadrants midway between the umbilicus and the anterior superior iliac spines below and the ninth costal cartilage above. Gentle suction is applied using a 2 or 5 ml syringe while the needle is moved about within the peritoneal cavity. The appearance and volume of the aspirate is noted and the material sent for biochemical and bacteriological analysis.

Normally less than 0.5 ml clear fluid can be aspirated. A positive result is obtained when the volume exceeds 0.5 ml or when the fluid is obviously abnormal. This suggests intra-abdominal disease. A negative paracentesis has no diagnostic significance. The technique is of value in the diagnosis of *acute intraperitoneal haemorrhage* as in acute pancreatitis when pure blood is aspirated that fails to clot. Paracentesis is especially helpful in the management of patients with non-penetrating abdominal injury. Alkaline bile-stained fluid, often containing food debris, is characteristic of a *perforated peptic ulcer*. The technique is not of value in the diagnosis of localized inflammatory disease.

The procedure is safe although the intestine may be accidentally penetrated when there are many adhesions or if there is a malignant peritonitis. This is usually readily appreciated from the appearance and microscopy of the aspirate.

Chylous ascites

The aspiration of an opalescent, cloudy fluid suggests the possibility of a chylous ascites which follows upon a leak of lymph into the peritoneal cavity. Chylous fluid contains absorbed fat (>5 mmol/l) in the form of particulate chylomicrons which floats on standing. This must be distinguished from pseudochylous ascitic fluid which is opalescent because it contains fat and granular material derived from degenerated cells (which tend to sediment). Chronic chylous ascites is associated with malignancy in 80% of cases. A wide variety of cases may underlie subacute chylous ascites.

PERITONEAL BIOPSY

Peritoneal biopsy is a most helpful technique for investigating unexplained ascites. It is simple and safe and is of particular value in the diagnosis of tuberculous peritonitis.

Method

The biopsy is obtained from the right or left lower quadrant lateral to the rectus sheath. A small area of the abdominal wall is anaesthetized using 1% procaine hydrochloride and the needle is introduced into the peritoneal cavity. It is advisable to discontinue the procedure if ascitic fluid is not aspirated readily. A small incision is made in the skin and the biopsy needle is introduced. When there is little fluid an assistant applies contralateral abdominal pressure to ensure the largest possible volume of fluid at the biopsy site. One or several portions of the peritoneum are taken from different quadrants of the same biopsy site, the Cope needle being suitable for obtaining more than one specimen. The needle is withdrawn and a tight dressing applied. The wound may be sutured if there is much ascites. The biopsy specimen is removed from the needle and placed in 10% formol-saline.

Types of needle

Side-biting, hook-type needles of the type described by Cope and Abrams are used. A Tru-Cut needle can be used but is less satisfactory.

Cope needle. This needle consists of a trocar, biopsy shaft and a snare. After penetrating the peritoneum the trocar is removed, ascitic fluid is aspirated for examination and the snare is introduced. The instrument is withdrawn until the snare engages the peritoneum. A biopsy is obtained by a forward-rotating advance of the biopsy shaft. The snare with the excized tissue is withdrawn and may be reinserted if further samples are required from a particular site.

Abrams needle. This needle comprises two concentric tubes. The outer tube has a short trocar point behind which is a deep notch which can be closed by the inner tube. The inner tube has a cutting edge. A spring clip holds a pin on the base of the inner tube in either the open or closed position. The needle is introduced with the notch in the closed position. The back hexagonal grip is twisted anticlockwise so that the notch is opened and a sample of the ascitic fluid is aspirated. When this is completed the needle is withdrawn until the notch is felt to engage the peritoneum. The outer tube is held steady and the back hexagonal grip is twisted sharply clockwise to pinch off a portion of peritoneum. The apparatus is withdrawn and the biopsy specimen is found either in the hollow point or inside the cutting cylinder.

Complications

It is unusual for peritoneal biopsy to be associated with any complication if the biopsy is performed when there is ascites. Haemorrhage or a leak of ascitic fluid can be prevented by a pressure dressing or by sutures.

PERITONEOSCOPY (LAPAROSCOPY)

This is a very useful technique for diagnosis of ascites because not only are the peritoneum and abdominal organs inspected, but biopsies can be obtained from the peritoneum and liver.

The procedure has been performed in humans since 1910. Despite this and its popularity in Europe and in the USA, it has not been widely used for the investigation of gastrointestinal disease in Britain.

Peritoneoscopy permits the visualization of the anterior surface of the liver, with the exception of the right lateral aspect, together with its leading edges and inferior surface. The anterior surface of the gallbladder and stomach can be seen, together with parts of the small bowel, colon and mesentery. The peritoneum over the diaphragm, anterior abdominal wall and falciform ligament are seen. The pancreas can be seen by lifting the left lobe of the liver. The pelvic organs (bladder, uterus, Fallopian tubes and ovaries) can be seen with the patient in the Trendelenburg position.

Method

Instruments

There are many forward- and oblique-viewing instruments, some with an operating channel for biopsy needles and probes. The fibreoptic light system is usually employed, and most instruments are insulated to permit diathermy. Instruments currently in general use are rigid, but flexible ones are being developed. The equipment consists of a trocar, sheath, telescope and light source. Air is insufflated through a Veress needle with retractable cannula, and this can be either via an automatic insufflator or a sterile sphygmomanometer bulb. Pre-warming in an oven or on an electrical pad, and use of an anti-fogging liquid on the lens are convenient. Cleaning should be followed by ethylene oxide or activated glutaraldehyde sterilization between cases.

Procedure

This is best performed on a table with full tilting facilities.

The patient is premedicated with an analgesic and a tranquillizer such as pethidine 50–100 mg and midazolam 8–10 mg i.v. with the procedure. Doses should be reduced in liver disease. General anaesthesia is an alternative, but this negates the advantage of peritoneoscopy over laparotomy.

The operator prepares by scrubbing, and wears gown and gloves as for major surgery. A puncture site is selected, avoiding epigastric vessels and visible collateral veins, abdominal scars and the falciform ligament.

The standard site is 2–4 cm inferior to the umbilicus in the midline. If better vision of the liver is needed then the puncture should be to the left of the midline above the umbilicus.

The skin and subcutaneous tissue are anaesthetized, as far as the parietal peritoneum if possible. A vertical incision is made to admit the trocar through the skin and fascia. The Veress needle is inserted through the wound and advanced carefully into the peritoneal cavity. When the tip is in place the needle is laid flat on the skin, and moderate distension of the abdomen with air or CO_2 is achieved (about 2–3 litres usually). The Veress needle is then removed and the peritoneoscope sheath (with trocar inserted) is passed into the peritoneum cavity. This requires force, and should be carried out with the table lowered and the arms of the operator extended fully to avoid sudden excessive penetration. When the peritoneal cavity has been entered the trocar is removed immediately. The sheath should be freely mobile when the telescope is passed. The room is darkened and the systematic inspection begins. It is important to remember that touching the falciform ligament and parietal peritoneum causes pain.

The liver, gallbladder, falciform ligament, parietal peritoneum and inferior surface of stomach and bowel should be inspected routinely. The spleen is seen only if enlarged. The pancreas may be seen with special manoeuvres. Pelvic organs can also be inspected if required.

When the examination is complete the telescope is removed, air allowed to escape and then the sheath removed. In ascites the peritoneal wound should be repaired, and in all patients the skin is closed with interrupted silk sutures.

The pulse and blood pressure are recorded at frequent intervals for 2–3 hours, and the patient kept in hospital overnight before discharge.

Complications occur in about 1–2% examinations, with an overall mortality of 0.03%. These deaths probably relate to liver biopsy, and the mortality is much lower than laparotomy. Problems which can arise include haemorrhage, bowel puncture, air embolism and puncture of an ovarian cyst.

Interpretation

The *cirrhotic* liver is nodular and in *hepatitis* the liver is red, swollen and shiny. A green liver is seen in *cholestatic* jaundice and various characteristics such as the state of the gallbladder and the liver edge have been claimed to help in the distinction between intra- and extrahepatic obstructive jaundice. Both primary and secondary *malignant disease of the liver* can be recognized. A *hepatoma* is often seen against the background of a cirrhotic liver and *metastatic nodules* are usually yellow-white and umbilicated. *Hydatid cysts* appear as characteristic pearly-white bulges.

Hydrops and fibrosis of the gallbladder can be identified. The peritoneum is dull and opaque in the presence of ascites. In *acute tuberculous peritonitis* it may be possible to see multiple millet seed-sized nodules surrounded by a halo of congestion. This appearance is very similar to that of metastatic malignant disease involving the peritoneum and the differentiation is usually made by biopsy and histological examination of a nodule. In *chronic tuberculous peritonitis* there are extensive adhesions, the nodules are confluent and the mesentery is contracted.

Indications

Liver disease. The inspection of the liver and targetted biopsy provides useful proof of diagnosis in alcoholic liver disease, macronodular as well as micronodular cirrhosis, hepatoma and metastatic carcinoma. Congenital cysts are usually readily recognized. Liver biopsy either by separate skin puncture or through the peritoneoscope can be used in patients with coagulation defects, because undue bleeding may be seen and controlled.

Ascites. Liver disease, peritoneal carcinoma or tuberculosis can usually be readily identified as causes. A forceps biopsy is practicable for the peritoneum but should be avoided for the bowel.

Portal hypertension. Dilated veins and splenic enlargement are seen.

Doubtful diagnosis of acute appendicitis. Especially in women this procedure may exclude unnecessary operations.

Identification of masses. Enlarged upper abdominal organs can usually be seen satisfactorily. Pelvic masses may also be seen and biopsied, but other abdominal masses are often obscured by bowel or omentum.

Others. Peritoneoscopy can be combined with cholangiography by either hepatic or gallbladder puncture and in this way assists in the diagnosis of *jaundice.* It is probably inferior to laparotomy or CT scanning in the staging of *lymphoma*, but can be used as a preliminary procedure in patients with serious abdominal complaints not explained by full medical investigation.

The procedure is unsatisfactory in marked obesity and after major abdominal surgery or peritonitis. It must be performed with caution when there are coagulation defects. Removal of fluid is required with tense ascites and hypovolaemic collapse and encephalopathy are hazards together with persistent leakage.

LAPAROTOMY

The use of exploratory laparotomy has rightly markedly decreased. Occasionally it still has a role in undiagnosed abdominal pain and in undiagnosed fever. In addition a full review of abdominal contents may supplement or alter diagnoses made prior to planned surgery.

References

Reynolds TB, Cowan RE. Peritoneoscopy. Chapter 26 in Wright R, Millward-Sadler GH, Alberti KLMM, Karrans. *Liver and Biliary Disease.* London, Bailliere-Tindall 1983
Paterson-Brown S, Thompson JN, Eckersley JRT, Pontint GA, Dudley HAF. Which patients with suspected appendicitis should undergo laparoscopy? *Br Med J* 1988; **296**: 1363 – 4

Further reading

Procedures

Drossman DA, *Manual of Gastroenterologic Procedures*. New York, Raven Press 1987

Cotton PB, Williams CB. *Practical Gastrointestinal Endoscopy*. Oxford, Blackwell Scientific 1982

Hunt RH, Waye JD. *Colonoscopy*. London, Chapman and Hall 1981

Ravenscroft MM, Swan CHJ. *Gastrointestinal Endoscopy and Related Procedures. (A handbook for nurses and assistants)*. London, Chapman and Hall 1984

Sellink JL, Miller RE. *Radiology of the Small Bowel (Modern Enteroclysis Technique and Atlas)*. The Hague, Martinus Nijhoff Publishers 1982

Bockus HL *et al*. *Gastroenterology. Volume one, Clinical Evaluation*. Philadelphia, Balliere Tindall 1985

Dagnini G. *Clinical Laparoscopy*. Padua, Piccin Medical Books 1980

Knill-Jones RP. A formal approach to symptoms in gastroenterology. *Clin Gastroenterol* 1985; **14**: 517–29

Grundy D, Read NW. Gastrointestinal neurophysiology. *Clin Gastroenterol* 1988; **2**: 1–258

Interpretation

Eastham RD. *Biochemical Values in Clinical Medicine*. Bristol, Wright 1985

Taylor KW. *Diagnostic Ultrasound in Gastrointestinal Disease*. Edinburgh, Churchill Livingstone 1979

Jones B, Braver JM. *Essentials of Gastrointestinal Radiology*. Philadelphia, WB Saunders 1982

Fishman EK, Jones B. *Computed Tomography of the gastrointestinal Tract*. Edinburgh, Churchill Livingstone 1988

Robinson PJA. *Nuclear Gastroenterology*. Edinburgh, Churchill Livingstone 1986

Scheuer PJ. *Liver Biopsy Interpretation*. London, Bailliere Tindall 1988

Talbot IC, Price AB. *Biopsy Pathology in Colorectal Disease*. London, Chapman and Hall 1987

Day DW, Husain OAN. *Biopsy Pathology of the Oesophagus, Stomach and Duodenum*. London, Chapman and Hall 1986

Reference text books

Bouchier IAD, Allan RN, Hodgson H, Keighley MRB. *Textbook of Gastroenterology*. London, Bailliere Tindall 1984

Sleisenger MH, Fordtran JS. *Gastrointestinal Disease*. Philadelphia, WB Saunders 1983

Wright R, Millward-Sadler GH, Alberti KGMM, Karran S. *Liver and Biliary Disease*. London, Bailliere Tindall 1985

Howat HT, Sarles H. *The Exocrine Pancreas*. London, WB Saunders 1979

Go VL, Gardner JD, Brooks FP, Lebenthal E, Di Magno EP, Scheele GA. *The Exocrine Pancreas*. New York, Raven Press 1986

Davenport HW. *Physiology of the Digestive Tract*. Chicago, Year Book Publishers Inc 1982

Bateson MC. *Gallstone Disease and Its Management*. Lancaster, MTP Press 1986

Allan RN, Keighley MRB, Alexander-Williams J, Hawkins C. *Inflammatory Bowel Disease*. Edinburgh, Churchill Livingstone 1983

Cooke WT, Holmes GKT. *Coeliac Disease*. Edinburgh, Churchill Livingstone 1984

Index